Alzheimer's, Depression and Dementia

A Husband's Observation

D. L. Bennett

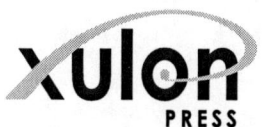

Copyright © 2008 by D. L. Bennett

Alzheimer's, Depression and Dementia
A Husband's Observation
by D. L. Bennett

Printed in the United States of America

ISBN 978-1-60647-744-1

All rights reserved solely by the author. The author guarantees all contents are original and do not infringe upon the legal rights of any other person or work. No part of this book may be reproduced in any form without the permission of the author. The views expressed in this book are not necessarily those of the publisher.

www.xulonpress.com

PREFACE

W*HY WAS THIS WRITTEN?* WHEN I STARTED IT WAS WITH THE IDEA OF A SHORT TIME JOURNAL FOR MY OWN USE FOR THE TIME OF HELEN'S ILLNESS. I NEVER EVEN CONSIDERED THE POSSIBILITY THAT IT MIGHT CONTINUE FOR A LONG TIME OR TILL THE DEATH OF MY WONDERFUL WIFE.

AFTER SEVERAL MONTHS I BEGAN TO WONDER IF IT WOULD BE HELPFUL, OR EVEN OF ANY INTEREST, TO OTHER PEOPLE. MY FIRST THOUGHT WAS THAT IT WAS SO PERSONAL I WOULD NOT WANT ANYONE TO READ IT.

THEN AFTER TALKING WITH SEVERAL FRIENDS, I DECIDED IT MIGHT BE WORTH CONSIDERING WHETHER IT SHOULD BE OFFERED AS A POSSIBLE HELP TO OTHERS. NOW, AFTER MORE THAN FIVE YEARS AND AFTER THE DEATH OF MY LOVING WIFE, I FIND IT HELPFUL FOR MY PERSONAL USE. MEMORIES FADE, OR AT LEAST MINE DOES. I CAN LOOK BACK AND SEE WHAT I WROTE ON CERTAIN DATES AND HAVE REASON TO BELIEVE IT IS ACCURATE.

MANY PEOPLE HAVE BEEN SO HELPFUL. I DO NOT DARE NAME A FEW BECAUSE I WOULD NOT BE ABLE TO NAME ALL OF THEM.

I HAVE A GREAT RESPECT FOR MANY PEOPLE IN THE MEDICAL PROFESSION. HOWEVER, I HAVE LEARNED THE HARD WAY THAT THEY ARE JUST AS HUMAN AS I AM. YOU WILL NOTICE THAT I WAS VERY DISAPPOINTED IN THE LACK OF CONCERN OF SOME PEOPLE IN THE MEDICAL PROFESSION. I MENTION CERTAIN THINGS, BUT I MAKE IT A POINT NOT TO GIVE THE NAMES OF ANY INDIVIDUALS OR ORGANIZATIONS.

D L BENNETT
OCTOBER 2007

I CAN BE REACHED AT:
TELEPHONE 501-922-2433
FAX 501-922-2469
E MAIL DLBENNETT01@YAHOO.COM

MAIL
33 SIERRA DR
HOT SPRINGS VILLAGE, AR 71909-3216

D L BENNETT

ALZHEIMER'S, DEPRESSION, AND DEMENTIA A HUSBAND'S OBSERVATIONS

By D L Bennett

I became aware of this problem June 25th, 2002 when we attended a meeting at Potter's Clay . Helen told a speaker she had heard what he read before. He said she could not have heard it because he only wrote it a few days before. There had been no major health problems for us during our marriage of almost 40 years. I was age 76 and she was 85 at the time.

We heard about the shooting at the LA airport about 3:00 PM July 4th. Helen thought she had heard about this a day or two before, and she "remembered" one man from Paris that they interviewed on TV. Then they said it had just happened. I did not realize how serious this was.

I got up at 4:00 AM July 10th to go to the bath room, and she told me she had chest pains. She chose not to call 911 or go to ER. She called me about 5:00. We called 911 and went to the ER. She said it was "a heck of a birthday present" for me. It was my birthday. She was in the hospital two days. The doctor told us one valve to her heart was smaller than it should be and that caused her heart to work harder. He said it was a choice between surgery and medication, and at her age he was afraid of surgery. She told me it sounded like the death sentence.

She woke about 2:30 AM July 28th and we went to the ER again. She was in the hospital three days that time.

Because of the things she could "remember" her regular physician said she had dementia. She knew what that is, and said she wished he had not said that. I do not remember ever hearing the word before.

She went to a ladies' meeting the night of August 8th. Normally she drives anywhere she wants to go. This time she asked me to take her. I took her and picked her up after the meeting. The next Sunday at Sunday school two ladies asked her about the meeting, and she could not tell them anything.

They knew something was wrong. After Sunday school she was so weak she had to go home. She asked me not to take her to the hospital and I honored her request. I went to a restaurant and bought two dinners which we ate at home.

We made an appointment with a nurse practitioner at the psychiatrist's office August 14th. She said she could see signs of Alzheimer's, and prescribed medications. We made an appointment with the psychiatrist for Aug. 28th.

The next Sunday she was not able to dress herself, so I dressed her and I prepared breakfast. We went out to eat about 1:00. She ate a good meal, but talked very little. She cried on the way home. We went to the 6:30 PM church service and she seemed OK till after the service when she was very tired and weak.

Friday night I stayed in her bed till about 4:30 when I went to my bed. We got up about 7:30, and I helped her dress. One other morning I found her sitting in her room sobbing after I had dressed. She could not talk with me. She took some medication and soon after that I found her in her room changing from her robe to a dress. At 9:05 I went to the living room and found her nicely dressed sitting in the chair she normally uses.

Flash back to the "tax season" of 1958. She had purchased a small house and rented out one room. She needed tax advise. A friend decided to recommend me, as well as do some match making. She did her own taxes the next four years. Now to August 1962. I went to a cafeteria and stood behind an attractive lady who told me I did her taxes a few years ago. We had dinner together and were married the following December 28th. We will soon celebrate the 40th anniversary of a wonderful marriage. We have no children.

Prior to our marriage her pastor advised her to tell me about her two breakdowns. One was at age 24 and the other at age 43, or about two years before. I told her I believed she had recovered and that I wanted to marry her. At this time I believe I made a wise decision.

Now back to 2002. After her sickness began she was not certain of her salvation in Christ. She was deeply concerned that she had not been a good Christian witness. We discussed several scriptures including John 6 and Second Peter where it says God is not willing that any should perish. At my suggestion she called her old friend Ruth, the widow of the pastor who married us. I called our pastor, Dr. Charles Long. He visited us and was a big help.

I told her I have read that people who have disappointments sometimes try so hard to forget them that they become buried so deep they do not even remember them, and these things must be dug out before they can be healed. I said I am afraid she has something like that. I told her it did not make any difference what it is, and that it would not make any difference in our marriage. We have had four or five talks this that.

We spent about an hour with our associate pastor, Elton Gray, August 10th. He was very understanding and helpful. On the way home I asked if she was now assured of her salvation in Christ. Her answer was a very definite yes. That was great news for me.

At 5:10 Wednesday she told me it was time to go the church dinner. We have had these Wednesday dinners for several years. I told her we do not have them now. I called a friend and confirmed they have been discontinued for the summer. We went out to eat. We went to a place we had eaten many times. She was unable to order for herself. She ate OK but it was a night to forget.

When we got home I took her in my arms before she sat down, and I talked about several things. I reminded her of what a great marriage we have had. Her eyes lit up like I had not seen in several days. We had a good conversation till we went to bed. That troubled look came back about 11:00 PM.

Thursday morning, August 22nd she seemed better when we got up. We went to the kitchen and she put the frying pan on to fry the eggs and meat. I walked out of the kitchen for five or ten minutes. I went back to the kitchen and found her looking at the frying pan as if she had no idea what to do. I finished getting breakfast and she ate about half what she usually eats for breakfast.

I called a friend of hers who is a retired nurse, and she insisted I get her where she could get help. Helen sat in the chair where she ate for more than an hour. Then at 9:45 I helped her to the couch where she sat till about 12:00 noon. I called the church and Pastor Long came over. Someone called the hospital. We got her to the hospital about 2:30 and she was admitted.

She has been silent for several days. Saturday, August 24th, she talked more and most of it was rational. Then in the afternoon she said it was time to meet them. I asked who we were to meet and she did not know, but she thought we had an appointment. Sometime that afternoon she said she felt like she was being forced to stay there.

Helen is a perfectionist. She accepted the job of church historian several years ago. One book she produced was lost by someone else after she delivered it to the church. Then she destroyed some records she thought she had on her computer. When she found she did not have them on her computer she was really upset. Our pastor and other people told her other people have records that can be used, and the church can go on even if we do not have the records she lost. No one blames her, but she cannot forgive herself.

In the spring of 2001 she got the idea to go into multi level sales with a food supplement company. Their products have made a great improvement in a serious back problem I had. The problem is we lost a considerable amount of money, and that bothers her. She says she put pressure on me to do it. That is true, but I have never blamed her. At age 76 I continue to do some work and I enjoy it. We live comfortably.

I attended church August 25th and did not visit her in the morning. When I got there in the afternoon she met me at the door and thought I was late. It was great to hear her voice again. She talked quite a lot till I left when visiting hours were over at 4:00. Her voice was not strong, but she was rational and I was on Cloud 9.

Monday, August 26th, I went to her room about 3:00 PM and found her asleep. I was careful not to wake her. I talked with the nurse about 4:00. The nurse said she had been asleep about two hours and if I did not wake her she would. She is a light sleeper. I kissed her lightly on the cheek and then held her hand. She looked very sad, and said nothing. About 5:15 the nurse and I put her in a wheel chair and took her to the dining area. I went out to eat and got back about 6:15. I was told she ate practically nothing. The nurse gave her some medication and told me she got Helen to eat some yogurt. She did not say one word to me today. I called about 9:00 PM and was told she talked some to the nurse who was asking some questions. The nurse said she gave yes and no answers. The next morning I called at 7:25 and the nurse said she did not sleep well. She attended the group meeting last night, and was up and down all night. She is not responding this morning.

I arrived at 3:15 and spent about an hour and a half with her in her room. She was very quiet. She knew who I was, but said practically nothing. She has never failed to know me or any other person she has known before. I went out to eat, and when I came back she had almost finished eating and was sitting at the table. She appeared to have eaten good. We stayed in the family room till I was told to leave at 7:35. One lady sitting at her table was talking very irrationally, and continuously. Helen told me she could not do anything to help that lady. That showed her concern for the other lady.

The next day I was able to see her just before 3:30. She was in the family room and was much better. I saw more smiles, heard more chuckles, and heard more talk than I have in two weeks. I felt great. We sat in the family room about an hour and then went to her room. I told her what the last two weeks had been like.

I met with the nurse manager. She went through a number of things in her files. There was very little I had not heard before:

A. time for the medication to get into her system.
B. She said they are set up for a treatment period of one to two weeks.
C. She said she expects Helen to go home in a week or two.

I got back to the family room about the time Helen finished eating. She appeared to have eaten a good meal. We had more heart to heart talk today than we have had since the problem began. I left about 7:15 PM.

The next morning I called about 6:50 and the social worker told me she had a good night and is still in bed. When I got there in the afternoon I was told she did not have a good night.

When I arrived about 3:30 she was sitting on the side of her bed almost in tears, and could not talk with me. Pastor Long came in a few minutes after I got there. She could not talk with him. I stayed till 5:30. One time she spoke one or two words I could understand. When I came back at 6:15 she had finished eating and was in the family room. We could not go to her room because they were waxing it, so we stayed in the family room till I was told to leave at 7:00. As I massaged her back I whispered something personal and she smiled briefly. The smile came and went in seconds.

I called about 7:30 AM August 30th and was told she had a good night's sleep. The nurse said she was eating breakfast, but was very silent. I got there about 3:30. She was in the family room and wore a smile. We talked quite a while and then went to her room. We closed the door to enjoy some privacy. The nurse opened the door and said it must stay open at all times so she could watch Helen. I said I would watch her. We closed the door about half way, got behind the door, and my wife and I embraced. The nurse invaded our privacy. Promptly at 4:30 the nurse told me visiting hours were over. I left and ate dinner. While I was outside waiting to get in another nurse and I talked about this incident.

Prior to the invasion of our privacy mentioned above Helen and I had a very serious conversation. She talked some and nodded her head a lot at what I said.

When I got back about 6:00 PM Helen was in the family room. A lady asked to speak to me outside in private. Much to my surprise a security guard was behind her. He said he heard I got quite loud outside today. I was shocked. After some quick thinking I asked if it was about 4:30. He said it could have been. I was accused of doing indecent things in public. After some quick thinking I told him it was not intercourse if that was what he meant. I was told very clearly there was no privacy in the hospital, and I was not permitted to embrace my wife till we got home. The remainder of the visiting period was not as nice as it was before the nurse invaded our privacy. I say without hesitation, reservation, or apology, that the action of these people drove my wife into deeper depression.

I called about 7:20 AM August 31st and was told she talked some to the staff. I arrived just prior to 10:00 AM. She was very attentive to my talk but said very little. She nodded her head to express approval of a number of things I said. Several times it appeared she was trying to talk with me but the words were just not understandable. I called at 9:05 PM and the nurse said the only words Helen had spoken to her were that the pills had gone down.

The next day I called about 7:00 AM and told a nurse about the security deal. The nurse said she would see me before visiting hours. When I got there about 9:40 the one I think of as the "mean nurse" said it was reported to her I was making a lot of noise in the hall. She did not say which hall. She walks the hall in the ward. She should know which hall it was. I had talked with another nurse in the hall, but I was not loud. She said it was reported to her, and she was the one who invaded our privacy. Does that make sense to you? I gave a handwritten report of the invasion of our privacy and the security deal to the security office.

I called Sept. 2nd about 7:20 AM and was told she slept last night, but is not talking this morning. Then they said she was eating at the time of the call. At 3:00 PM our deacon and I had an interesting interview with the social worker. We discussed her medications, etc. He said the doctor sees families on Thursdays and Tuesdays nearing release. He seemed receptive to my objection to the hospital's actions in the security deal. He said the nurse manager would call me and discuss this. The nurse manager and I talked later.

Helen talked very little today and was very low about 3:30. One nurse really tried to help. Just before I left I asked if she wanted to go to the family room. She said if we went there we would get in trouble again—obviously referring to the security deal. I called at 9:05 PM and was told she answered some questions at the meeting tonight, but only gave direct answers and nothing was volunteered.

I called at 7:23 AM Sept. 3rd and was told there was no change. I talked with a nurse about 9:00 about the incident, and she said another nurse would talk with me. She said the report I was loud caused her to call security. I tried to reason with her, but she said to calm down or leave. She said Helen seems to be more nervous when I am there than when I am not there. I did not tell her, but I do not believe her. I found Helen to be very silent, and she looked very sad. As soon as visiting hours were over I gave a report of the security deal to a lady security officer.

The nurse manager called me at 10:30 AM. I asked if she had read my note. She said she had, but did not seem to know what it was. We agreed I would be there at 3:00 today. She claimed nurses reported to her Helen and I have been too affectionate, including in the family room. I said a man and his wife should be allowed some privacy. She said to keep the doors open at all times. I said when security was called it should have been done so neither Helen nor the public knew about it. She said it could have been done another way. I said it should have been done another way. She said it could have been done another way. She said she would bring it up at a meeting. I did not tell her, but bringing it up at a meeting may prevent it happening again, but it will do nothing about the harm it did to Helen.

At my request the nurse manager went to Helen's room to talk with her about the security deal. She spent about five or six minutes and said she would come back. Helen was just not able to talk with her. At 7:00 PM, the end of the visiting period, Helen was really "out of it"—not in the real world. I tried to help her walk to the family room after taking her to her room in a wheel chair. It was difficult for her to walk. An employee helped me get her to the family room and then I left. Earlier in the day she had walked a little more. Pastor Long said she talked with him more today than she had recently. I called about 9:25 PM and was told she responded a little at the meeting, and she was in the family room watching TV.

I called early September 4th and was told they had trouble getting her to bed the night before, and did not think she slept any. She was in the breakfast room then. I demanded to talk with the doctor. I strongly expressed my dissatisfaction with the security deal and said I have seen a definite deterioration in her condition since that time. I said the sooner she gets out of that place the better. I was told the doctor would call me about 8:30.

During the time she was there I was not permitted to talk with the doctor.

As I entered about 3:30 the nurse told me she had a good day till shortly before I got there when she had direa and her blood pressure dropped. I found her on the bed. Even though her eyes were open she seemed to be asleep or just "out". She soon recognized me and said she was in a fog. She did not know where she was. I told her I would be honest with her. I said she had a spell like she had in 1960. I explained she had been at the hospital 13 days. She was very weak and talked very little. For the most part I just remained with her and kept silent. About 4:30 a nurse told me a lady doctor wanted to see her alone. I went to the lobby. I then went to the cafeteria and was back at her room at 6:00. She was in the family room. She asked if she saw the lady doctor. I checked with the nurse and was told the lady doctor did see her. I was told the nurse manager would see me tomorrow.

We stayed in the family room quite a while, and then walked to her room. She was very weak, but stood at the door of her room ten or fifteen minutes. I finally got her to sit in a chair and pulled the chair into the room with her sitting on it. She sat there quite a while and then got up and stood awhile. Then she sat on the side of the bed. A nurse told me she ate about 25% of her dinner. I called about 9:30 PM and was told she was still up. The nurse said she had to practically force her to bed last night and she got to sleep about 3:00 AM. She said she plans to let her go to bed when she wants to tonight.

The next morning I called and was told she got to bed about 10:00 and got a good night's sleep. When I got there about 3:25 she was in the family room and was very weak. She spoke very little. When I got back about 6:00 she was in the family room. A nurse told me she ate almost half her breakfast but only about 8 bites of lunch. The nurse spoon fed her. She ate some of her dinner. She ate very little of the turkey which looked good. She ate all the potatoes in the potato soup but left the juice. She spoke very little and was very weak. I called at 9:52 and was told she is still in the family room watching TV. She is not saying a lot, but did take her medication.

When I called the next day a nurse said she went to bed late but slept. I expressed my deep concern about her staying there any longer. I insisted on talking with the nurse manager sometime today other than visiting hours. The nurse insisted Helen had improved since going there but would not comment on her decline the last six days. I know the reason, and I am sure she did too.

I got to her room about 3:40 and found her asleep. I "watched her sleep" till about 4:40. Normal noise does not wake her. After an hour and five minutes I spoke to a nurse as I walked out. My voice woke her. She said a few words in a more normal voice than I had heard since she had been there. I got back about 6:00. They had what looked like a good meal. She ate about half her meat and said she was too full. I encouraged her to go to her room with me. It was very difficult for her to walk even with my help. She talked quite a bit and her voice was stronger than in recent days, but not as strong as when she first woke. She smiled occasionally. I called at 9:30 PM and the nurse told me her regular physician ordered an MRI. She said Helen seemed better than when I left.

I called about 8:45 AM September 7th and was told she was eating and that she slept well the night before. She will have an MRI at 12:15. I went in about 10:00 and someone was doing her hair. She was silent, but did speak a few words to me. She seemed very weak. She ate a cup of ice cream. I spoon fed her a few bites and then she ate it by herself. I left about 11:30. When I came back she had her lunch tray, but had eaten practically nothing. I spoon fed her one bite of the burger meat, but she would not eat it. She ate most of her green beans as I spoon fed her. That was all she ate after I got there and she had eaten very little, if anything, before I got there. After giving up on her eating more I pushed her back to her room in the wheel chair. A new doctor who seemed nice came in about 4:10. She answered most of his questions, but could not tell him her occupation or where she worked. I answered those questions. I called about 10:00 PM and the nurse said she had been really quiet tonight and was then in bed.

A nurse called me at 7:20AM Sept. 8th and said Helen got up at 1:00 AM to go to the bath room and fell and broke her left wrist. She said I could get in as soon as I got there. I got there at 9:00 AM just as the doctor arrived. The doctor said the break was slight and it would be sore a month or so. A nurse said Helen had talked with her more since the fall than she talked all day yesterday. Her hand was quite blue, but she said the pain was slight. She spoke very clearly and her voice was almost normal and fairly strong. I left at 11:00 and went back at 2:00. I woke her at 4:15 to tell her I was going to the church picnic. I called at 9:40 PM. The nurse said she fed herself tonight and she ate fairly well. She is having a snack now and is talking more. PRAISE THE LORD.

I called at 7:23 AM September 9th. The nurse said Helen slept well and did not need anything for pain. I got there about 3:00 and talked with the social worker. He gave me some information about nursing homes and med-i-care. He said he would consult our insurance and med-i-care and get back with me. When I saw her she was very silent all the hour or so I was there. We stayed in the family room. She did not want to go to her room. When I got back at 6:00 it was about the same. When I told her about my brother's surgery she seemed to understand, but was unable to talk.

I called at 7:45 AM September 10th and they put Helen on the phone. Her voice was weak, but she talked quite a bit. It was great to hear her voice. I got there about 3:00 and talked with a man from the Department of Human Services. While I was talking with the social worker Helen walked by being assisted by staff. Then we met the social worker in the family room. He left it up to us to decide whether Helen goes to a nursing home. She could not talk with him. I estimate she ate something over a third of her dinner. I was told she ate 90% of her breakfast and lunch. As we walked to her room she had difficulty walking, but not as much as she has had before. When we got there we found her closet door was open as well as two or three drawers where her clothes are kept. A male patient walked in behind us and asked if that is where the gifts are. I had not seen him before today. He walked into her room at least twice after that before I left. Most of her clothes and personal things were laying on her bed. When I reported it a nurse agreed to have it investigated. I left shortly after 4:00. When I called at 9:50 PM I was told she talked when she took her medication and she was then in the family room watching TV. I asked about the clothing deal mentioned above and was told they are not sure what happened. The nurse said "we watch all of them".

I called at 7:27 September 11th and a nurse said she slept well and is talking. The nurse said they were eating then and suggested I call at 11:00. I called again at 11:00 and was told I could pick her up and take her home. I got there about 12:00 and she was very quiet. I forgot to take a suitcase and the nurse put her things in a plastic bag. It took at least five minutes to get her to sit down in a wheel chair. The nurse was to take her to the lobby while I got the car. When I got back to the lobby I called to see why she was not there. I was told Helen had decided she wanted to stay there. In my opinion she had decided she needed more care than we could provide at home. I believe it was a good decision. I talked with her about going to a nursing home. She remained very silent. I told her she needed to get out of that place. I left about 4:40. I called later and a nurse said "she's fine. She's asleep".

I called at 7:20 AM September 12th and was told she got a good night's sleep. She said I could call between 11:00 and 12:00 and talk with Helen. I called about 12:00 and talked with Helen. Her voice was very weak. I told her I would see her about 2:00. I was mixed up on the visiting hours which started at 3:30. When I got there I had to wait. I met the social worker at 3:00. He told me about the BOCK test. She was very quiet. I pushed her to her room in a wheel chair. One time she said "I just don't understand the reason". She was very understanding and agreed when I mentioned our long and happy marriage. I left about 4:40. When I got back about 6:00 she was at the table and had eaten about half her food by herself. I spoon fed her the ice cream. I took her to her room in the wheel chair. We talked some and both of us were near tears. I talked about her going to a nursing home and she did not comment. The social worker said she told him she would go.

I called at 9:02 and was told she talked a lot at the meeting. I called at 7:52 the next morning and was told she slept very little, but is talking some. The nurse said she seemed to be afraid to go to sleep.

Back to September 6th. The nurse manager called me as I had requested. She said the lady doctor found her impaired in several ways:

1. The doctor was not able to complete because of lack of response.
2. Helen is impaired in several ways:
   A. Construction—putting things together—mildly.
   B. Verbal response.

They recommended having 24 hour a day care. The nurse manager expects her to be released some time next week. She said I could get her medical records by signing a release. The next day I arrived about 3:20. She talked very little and we stayed in the family room all the time. She did not want to go to her room. I left at 4:47 and when I got back about 6:00 I found she had eaten practically nothing. I tried to spoon feed her but she refused to eat. A nurse said she ate 25% of her breakfast and 50% of her lunch. The lady from the BOCk test said she answered three pages of questions and then suddenly stopped. The BOCk lady called me at home and asked a few questions she refused to answer. One was whether we had any children. A friend not connected with the hospital said she probably got tired of looking at a piece of paper. During the 6:00 to 7:00 visit we had a serious conversation even though I did most of the talking. She seemed to understand and agree with me. Even in the family room we had enough privacy at times to talk quietly and seriously. I left at 7:05. I called at 10:06 PM and was told she talked very little tonight, but she did have a good day. The nurse was trying to get her to take her medicine when I called.

I called at 8:06 AM September 14th and was told she is talking more this morning. I arrived at 10:00 and she was in the family room. She talked quite a bit and her voice was not quite as weak. We stayed in the family room till I was told to leave at 11:00. I helped her walk to her room. She was weak, but stronger than a few days ago. She appeared to want to go back to the family room and I helped her go back. A nurse said it was time for me to go and she would help Helen. I got back at 1:55 and a nurse said Helen had been asleep ten or fifteen minutes. She slept another fifty or fifty-five minutes without waking. We talked briefly and she went back to sleep. Shortly after 4:00 I woke her to say I had to go and would see her about 10:00 tomorrow. I called at 10:05 PM and they told me she was already asleep.

I called at 7:41AM September 15th and was told she is talking more this morning. At 9:55 AM I entered her room and found her sitting on the side of her bed with her feet on the floor. One shoe was on her foot and the other nearby on the floor. She was very silent. After about five minutes I asked if her wrist hurt. She said it did not hurt much and then there was more silence. I left shortly after 11:00 AM. I was back at 2:00 and we spent considerable time in the family room. The staff brought in a tray of bananas, oranges, plumbs, grapes, cookies, and two kinds of cheese. She did not reach for any of this. I hand fed her some grapes and two pieces of cheese. She also ate most of two cookies. A nurse helped me walk her back to her room. She talked to me a very little. Associate Pastor Elton Gray came in just before 4:00. She spoke two sentences to him very clearly. That was the most I had heard her say today at one time. I called at 9:40 PM and was told she was talking some and ate some ice cream with her medication, and that she ate about 50% of each meal today.

I called at 9:40 AM September 16th and was told she slept fairly well and she is fairly quite. I arrived at 3:20 and she was in the family room. We stayed there quite awhile and then I helped her walk to her room. She spoke very few words before I left at 4:30 when the nurse told me to go. I was back at 5:55 and a nurse said wait till they finished eating . I stayed in her room and when I went to the family room she had eaten practically nothing. I spoon fed her till she had eaten practically all the food on her tray except the apple sauce and bread. She did not drink much, if any, of the milk, tea, or cola. She did not drink any of it after I got there. I called at 9:20 PM and was told she was about the same as when I left. Then I was told a nurse is with her trying to get her to bed.

TO THE NURSING HOME

I called about 7:35 AM September 17th and was told she is talking some. Her voice is still weak. When a nurse went to her room this morning Helen was standing at the sink in the bathroom, and was able to wash, comb her hair, etc. I arrived at the hospital at 3:25 PM. When the door was opened there was Helen in the wheel chair with her hospital possessions ready to leave. NO ONE at the hospital had told me she was leaving. A nurse was on one side and a lady from the nursing home was on the other side of the wheel chair. The nursing home lady told me she was taking Helen in her van. I told her Helen was going in my "van". I have a telephone recorder at home and it was turned on. When I got home there was no message. The hospital just DID NOT bother to tell me they were taking my wife to the nursing home. She rode with me to the nursing home. She talked very normally while we drove to the "home". It was great to be with her in a normal sitting, and to hear her voice again. After we checked in at the business office and went to her room she said something to the effect it was a mistake to leave the other place. About 7:15 PM she mentioned something she needed from home and I went home and got it for her.

I called the next morning about 8:00 and was told she was disorientated. I went down about 1:30 and a lady doctor was seeing her at that time. She seemed to be having one of those bad days I have seen so often. I went to the business office and left some things they had requested. When I went to her room she was sleeping.

The next day she was very sad, but I got her to move around a little on a walker. In tears she said she would hate for anyone to see her in that condition. A nurse showed us a room where we could have some privacy and we spent about ten minutes there. A very nice nurse took me out and talked with me while she was in therapy. After therapy I took her to her room on a walker. We stood in the door several minutes, and then she got in the wheel chair. They encouraged her to go to the dining room to eat. The speech therapist asked to sit at her table to see if she had trouble swallowing. I left at 12:00 and was back at 6:15. A nurse told me it takes a few days to get adjusted. I do not see how anyone could ever get adjusted to a nursing home. They are necessary, and I believe the staff tries to do a good job. But patients have problems and get confused about doctor appointments, etc. It spreads to other people. I helped her prepare for bed before leaving about 9:00 PM.

She talked quite a bit the next day, but was somewhat confused about a doctor's appointment. A couple came to visit and she was able to talk with them in a normal way. I took two of her paintings and hung them on her wall. I helped her walk on a walker and then put her in the wheel chair and pushed her to the dining room.

I was told they were moving her to another room. When I learned who the room mate would be I objected because I knew the case. The patient did not know anyone—even her husband. They did not move her. Then they told me they were moving her to another room with a 93 year old lady who was also an artist. Her daughter visits often and she too is an artist. Several of her paintings are on the wall. It did not take long to learn the room mate tries to rule the roost— including telling the staff and me exactly what to do.

Helen and I went out to lunch September 24th. I asked where she wanted to go and she said I mentioned the Panda. I had mentioned it, but she did not reply. We went to the Panda and then to her doctor's appointment. Then we drove to De Gray Park.

The next day we had an appointment with her Chiropractor. He was very understanding, and said I should take her out as often as possible. We went back to our house about 9:25 and were there till about 3:00. It was great to be at home together again, but it was also difficult because I am sure she, as I, wondered if we would ever be back there again as in the past.

When I got there the next day she was sitting on the side of the bed. She looked at me, but said nothing at that time. Bud and Gertrude came and she hardly spoke to them. After they left I took her outside in a wheel chair. We sat on the porch about an hour. I said I was going out to eat and then to the church. Her lips said nothing, but her eyes said it all. She did not want me to leave, and I stayed with her. When her meal was brought out I do not think she would have eaten anything if I had not been there. I spoon fed her, and she ate practically all of what looked like a good meal. At about 7:00 when I told her I was leaving she was practically in tears.

When I got there September 26th she had eaten practically none of her lunch. I spoon fed her and she ate practically all of it. Bette, a close friend of hers, came and I walked out so they could talk in private. When Bette left I went back in and she was almost in tears, and very silent. When her dinner was brought in I spoon fed her again. When I left she was near tears. I was too, but I think she showed it more than I did. We have both cried a lot—both together and separately.

When I arrived September 27th her tray was before her but she had eaten very little. I spoon fed her and she ate most of her meal. I took her outside in the chair. I mentioned tomorrow's church dinner to her and she said very little. When her dinner was brought in I spoon fed her some and then she took the fork and fed herself. When I left she was in tears.

I could see no difference September 28. I talked with her about the church dinner and got no response. About 5:30 I took her to the car in the wheel chair. When I started to help her in the car she started crying. I took her back in. When she finished eating I went to the church dinner alone. I saw her September 29th after church and lunch. There was no noticeable difference.

I got there about 7:00 AM September 30th. When she woke her voice was weak, but more like it had been for years when she first woke in the morning. I sat by her bed a few minutes and then she got up and I dressed her. Then she went back to her silence and sad look. We went to a doctor's office to have her wrist examined. We met a friend there and I could hardly talk to her.

After an appointment with her regular physician October 1st we got to our home about 11:00. We drove into the garage, but she was unable to get up the steps into the house. We went out to lunch and she ate a good meal. Then to the pharmacy to get a prescription filled. Every time I turned toward Hot Springs she cried. I drove to the church where we met with the associate pastor who was very helpful. He volunteered to go to the nursing home with us and then I took him back to the church.

She talked a little more. I said something about having five days like this. In surprise she said "five days?." I assured her that was correct. I got her on the walker. She walked very little, but that helped. She was very low and talked very little October 2nd.

The next day she said, with no prompting from me, that due to her having trouble standing on her feet she would not be able to do what she wanted to do even if she went home. I agreed with her. We agreed it would be wonderful to have her home again. Later she said she felt like her brain had been sterilized. Just after saying that she laughed, and I laughed too. That was the first time we had laughed in many days. I told her I do not know how to "unsterilize" her brain, but since she said it that way I believe her brain is coming back. I went home thinking she was making improvement.

The following day I took her outside on a walker. She asked where our car was and I showed it to her. She said that was not ours. We went closer and she agreed it was our car. I mentioned eating out. She said she needed her purse if we were going to the car. She said nothing about going our to eat. When we got to the restaurant she said she wished we had not come. I think she was embarrassed to be seen on a walker. She ate a good meal.

I arrived about 1:00 October 5th and spoon fed her again. When her dinner was brought out she said "oh no" again as if there was too much food. I spoon fed her again and she ate almost all of it. Bette visited again and then told me she believes Helen is improving because she answers in whole sentences.

I was invited to have dinner with friends after church October 6th so I did not see her till 3:15. She woke when I got there and talked very little. She had difficulty with bladder control as soon as they brought in her tray. She always cries from embarrassment when that happens. When I left I took some of her clothes with me to wash, and she was upset because of some things I took. I did not understand why she was upset. I took them home to wash.

She talked very little October 7th. I got there after they picked up her lunch tray and was told she ate about half her lunch. When they brought her dinner tray she was almost in tears, and said she could not eat all that. I spoon fed her and she ate most of it. A few minutes after they took her tray out she said she did not know where we could go to eat. I said I hated to tell her, but she had just eaten. I asked if she wanted to go out tomorrow and she did not reply. She was in tears when I left at 7:00.

Pastor Long visited October 8th as did Raymond and Lillian. She was glad to see them, but had very little to say. I went out to get protective underwear and she did not want me to do that because she hates to wear them. When the dinner tray was brought in she acted like that was too much and was almost in tears. I spoon fed her and she ate everything except a piece of white bread. She prefers wheat bread. An aid said she would ask the kitchen to give her wheat bread in the future. I left her in tears at 7:00 and went back to an empty house. The next day was about the same routine. When I spoon fed her she ate like she was hungry.

The physical therapist told me she has gotten where she will not cooperate with therapy, and without her cooperation they can do nothing for her. I got her on the walker and she walked quite a distance to the beauty shop. I made an appointment for her, but she showed no interest. When the tray was brought out it was the old routine. I told her she cannot live without eating. She ate a good part of her meal.

With my help she ate most of her meal October 10th. She will often start with the fruit, which they serve often, and then eat meat and other food later. When I left at 7:00 we were both in tears. I told her I had to get some food and rest. I know the Lord is our only hope, and he is faithful. She may never be home again, but the Lord could perform a miracle. I believe it was Job who said "The Lord gives, and the Lord takes away. Blessed be the name of the Lord".

The speech therapist called me October 11th and said Helen is not cooperating with her and she may have to drop her. That is similar to what the physical therapist said. When I got there a little before 1:00 a very understanding employee was spoon feeding her. She ate quite a bit, but nothing like all her lunch. She talked a little, but did not smile all day. When dinner was brought in she ate quite a bit of it as I spoon fed her. She did not have a kidney accident today. A nurse said she is taking medicine for that but sometimes it takes a month or so for that to work. It seems to be working now after about 17 days. After she had eaten, a little before 7:00, I told her I had to go eat and then go home, and she started crying. It was hard to leave her crying and then go "home" alone.

Many people have been so helpful. Gene and Helen A. have been so helpful. Gene, a retired military man, told me his first wife had problems very similar to Helen's. He took some time off to be with her before her death.

Helen and I have trusted Christ for many years. Looking back it seems we have failed in many ways, but He is faithful. I know many people who have had problems similar to what we have now. It was so easy to go our own way. Now I know what they faced. We realize we could not provide the care she needs if she were home. The nursing home cannot make that place home no matter how hard they try. And they do try. My personal desire is that the Lord will take her home first and then take me in a short time—maybe two months. That is probably just a cowardly and selfish desire on my part, and I do not say what He will do.

As of October 13th her kidneys are under control, but it continues to be necessary to help her to the bathroom and that is so embarrassing to her. I spoon fed her today.

October 14th. She could not believe it was Monday because she did not go to church yesterday. We discussed her not going to church because she was confined to the nursing home.

The next day she talked some, but could not carry on normal conversations. She just said brief sentences. I pushed her wheel chair to the front of the building and she said I was too pushy. (no pun intended). She said she wished she had an ice cream cone or something. That was the first time she had asked for anything of that sort since she had been sick. I said I would go get her one and she did not want me to go out. I pushed her to the nurse's station, and said we were going out. She did not want to go out. I went out and came back with two double dip cups of ice cream. I did not need to spoon feed her. We went out in the sun and she seemed to enjoy it. Sandy, our pastor's wife, came to visit and Helen enjoyed talking with her. When her tray was brought in she said she had eaten too much already. I spoon fed her and she ate less than half her food. After I gave up she picked up the fork and ate a few bites of her peas, carrots, and macaroni. I left at 6:45 and told her I was going to eat and to the store. She cried. She was also displeased that I took some of her clothes to wash. Could that be because she previously did the laundry? I hardly knew how to turn on the washer.

The next day when I went in about 2:00 her lunch tray had been taken out. She was very sad and unwilling to go outside. When her dinner tray was brought in she ate less than usual. When I left a little before 7:00 I think it was more difficult to leave than it had ever been.

She had an appointment with a nurse practitioner October 17th and was able to talk very little there. After the appointment we went to the Panda for lunch. It was very difficult to get her out of the car and into the restaurant where she ate not more than half a regular meal. Then back to the nursing home, where I was told that due to her refusal to do therapy med-i-care would not pay. I tried to discuss this with her, but never was certain whether she understood.

When I got home I called Helen A. who said Helen's case is so similar to her mother's, and her mother died at age 88. My Helen is 85. We have discussed our hope in Christ many times, but it continues to be a difficult time.

She talked some October 18th, but less than a few days ago. She knows everything that is going on, but is just unable to express in words what she wants to do. She pressed her arms on the chair and I thought she wanted to walk. I was right. She walked on the walker as I helped her. I spoon fed her at noon and at 6:15.

Sunday she talked very little and walked ten or twelve feet with my help and without the walker. I spoon fed her. The next day she talked some, but her voice was so low I could hardly understand her. She walked some on the walker. I had to take her to the bathroom four times between 1:00 and 7:00.

The next day I talked with a new psychologist recommended by the home about the possibility of his seeing her. Dr Josef gave me some good advise about this.

Today was not a lot different. She was quiet, talked very little, and I spoon fed her.

When she did talk October 23rd it was so low I could not understand a lot of it. She did cooperate with the physical therapist. At 3:30 I insisted she go to bed and she slept about two hours.

The next day we saw her chiropractor. On the 20 mile trip the only thing she said that I could understand was that the sun was bright. We went by our house, but she was unable to get up the steps from the garage. I spoon fed her lunch when we got back to the nursing home. When they brought out the evening meal I spoon fed her till I thought she would eat no more. When I started to take out the tray she objected. I waited awhile, and then she ate most of the macaroni and cheese. I was thankful I waited because she had eaten so little. When I left about 7:00 I told her I would see her tomorrow afternoon. She said very clearly "oh no, not that long".

She walked some on the walker with me helping her. The physical therapist came up then and took her for regular therapy. I asked if Helen "passed" the therapy and she said she did. I asked Helen about Linda Josef, Phd going to see her and she did not reply. So I said she would. When I got home I called Dr Josef.

Helen A. called me October 26th. She and Gene have been so helpful. We discussed Helen's condition as well as mine. I told her the church has a record of who to call in case of emergency—our family and attorney.

After church October 27th two Sunday school classes got together for a barbeque dinner. Bev prepared a plate for me to take to Helen and one for me to take home. When I got to the "home" Helen's tray was before her but she had eaten so little. When I got home I called Charles whose wife is in a nursing home. We had a lengthy conversation.

I could see no change October 28th. I called her regular physician and requested that he evaluate her medication and see if any changes should be made.

I asked Helen twice if she had any visitors this morning, and she did not reply. I was really asking if Dr Josef saw her. Dr Josef called me and said she saw Helen. She quoted Helen as saying her confusion started in January. I had not noticed any change at that time. Dr Josef said she was not experienced with people who have Helen's type of problems. She strongly recommended prayer. I told her a lot of people are praying for her and me. The new psychologist recommended certain changes in her medication that appear to be helpful.

I went to the nursing home about noon October 29th and told Helen I was going to Little Rock to get information from the Med-i-care office. When I returned about 5:30 she had been taken to the hospital with what they thought was a possible stroke. I called our pastor and then went to the hospital. There I was told it was dehydration. For some time she has refused to drink much liquids even though the staff and I have encouraged her to drink more. Could it be she is afraid more liquids will cause more bladder problems? She talked with me more October 31st than she has in some time but it was not much today. She was fed by IV. Then they brought in some broth and semi solids November 1st. She ate quite a bit of it, but refused the remainder.

They brought in some soft food November 2nd and she ate very little. A doctor said she seems to be improving, and her sodium is normal. He mentioned the possibility of a feeding tube, but I got the impression he did not think that would be necessary.

I got there in time to feed her lunch November 3rd, and she ate very little. I was told she ate very little breakfast. She slept most of the time between 3:00 and 4:00. The doctor, whom I knew, came in about 4:00. I followed him out to the hall and asked what he thought. He said something about four to six weeks and then letting her go. I asked if that meant she would be dead before the first of the year, and he said that was right. Then he said he had been wrong before.

As soon as I got back in the room she said something to the effect she heard our conversation. I had followed the doctor outside hoping she would not hear. I did not repeat what he said, but I have no doubt she heard it all. We talked about the security we have in Christ and the hope we have for eternity with Him. She looked concerned, but was not in tears. We both seemed to be confident of our hope in Christ. These are serious times, but we can be thankful for His mercy. She was transferred to the nursing home part of the hospital November 5th.

November 6th she acted so strange I called a nurse who decided she was hungry. She brought in some pudding and apple sauce. After a few bites she went to sleep. She would not eat dinner. I talked with a nurse who said she would work with her. I left early because I just could not stand to see her in that condition.

The next day when her lunch was brought in she ate without being spoon fed. She probably ate more for lunch than she ate all day yesterday. Shortly after eating lunch she went to sleep, and slept till 5:30 when they brought in her tray. She ate practically nothing for dinner.

She would not eat at noon November 8th. They put in a feeding tube that afternoon and I was told they would feed her through that beginning with the evening meal. As of November 9th I could see no difference except they fed her through the tube.

Carol told me there were 39 days when his wife could not talk with him. It has been 81 days since Helen has been able to carry on a normal conversation with me. When I went to her room after church she spoke to me. Just one word and nothing more at that time. About two hours later she asked if I went to church. There was very little change November 11th.

She was taken back to the nursing home Nov. 12th as I had been told. I got there shortly after she did. She had visitors from the church in the afternoon. We talked very little before she went back to sleep.

She said she did not like the looks of the stand that holds the feeding tube. She talks with me a little more and I am told she talks a little more with others when I am not there. I talked with a nurse in her regular physician's office who quoted the doctor as saying Helen would never get any better. It is so sad to see her in that condition. However, it did not disturb that idiot who calls herself a nurse. She ended the conversation by saying "have a nice day" and hung up before I could respond.

When I went in November 18th she told me in a clear, understandable voice a lady in the business office wanted to see me. This was the most words, and the clearest, I had heard in several weeks. Later she asked if I ever drive the van—our second car. I told her I drive the van just enough to keep it in shape. I did not tell her I had put it on the lot for sale. I asked if she thought we needed two cars and she did not reply. I changed the subject. Then she mentioned a friend she worked with whom we expected to call. She said something about wishing she could be normal and go home. This is the best conversation we have had since she got sick. It is wonderful.

Her psychologist came in about the time I got there November 19th. I could see nothing interesting about what he did or about the results. After he left the remainder of the day was about like those days before the wonderful day yesterday.

The next day was about "normal". I left about 5:30 because she was asleep and did not appear to know I was there. I got there about 12:35 November 21st and found her sitting in the wheel chair. She appeared to be very tired. It was obvious she had an accident and they had not changed her sheets. After getting back from therapy at 3:00 she went to bed and was asleep very quickly. Since she was asleep I left early again.

November 22nd has been about like the last three days. The day before that was so wonderful. Recently I saw a headline in thee Village Voice that said "One is a Lonely Number." I did not read the article. The headline said it all. The next day I went in about 1:30 and they had just changed her bed. They did it two more times in about an hour. Then she went to sleep. When she woke she said something to the effect she would never get out of this place. I did not tell her she would, but I encouraged her that it was a possibility. I told her if she did not we both belong to the Lord and he will care for both of us. She seemed to agree, but said very little. She went to sleep again. Her eyes opened a few times, but not for long. I left about 5:45 to eat. Then to the office and then to an empty house.

When I went in November 24th they told me the feeding tube causes more kidney action. After being changed twice she went to sleep. When she went to the nursing home I took several newspapers and magazines which she read at home. She showed no interest in reading them. Today her roommate offered us her newspaper as she always does. I read part of it and laid it on her bed. She picked it up and read for a few minutes. I went to the car and got one of her favorite magazines which I had ready just in case she showed any sign of wanting it. She took it and read for twenty or twenty-five minutes. I asked about what she read. She said she did not like what she read about some of the things they are doing to Israel. I said we should not be surprised at that. She said the U S Government is spending so much money helping Israel's enemies. We discussed this briefly. Then she started reading again. Her reading time and our discussion lasted about forty minutes. She went to sleep about 4:00 or 4:30 and slept till 5:45.

I took the Campus Crusade magazine in the next day. She read some of it and we discussed what she read. Conversations two days in a row—that was great. Her reading and our conversation lasted about fifty minutes. Soon after that a young man came in to give her therapy. That disturbed her till she was near tears, and that ended our conversation.

She had an appointment November 26th to have a video of her swallowing. She was concerned about not having proper clothes, thought she was late, and wondered how she would get on the van to get there. I told her the van was built to accommodate people with problems, and it was the nursing home's responsibility to get her there on time. When she got back I got her on the walker a short time. Then the therapist came in. When he finished she was really tired.

People at the church and other places have been so helpful. Four different groups invited me to eat Thanksgiving dinner with them. I accepted the one with Jim and Ann, a couple we have been close to a long time. It was difficult to leave Helen alone. What would I do without the scriptures and the prayers of other believers?

I had Thanksgiving dinner with Jim and Ann as planned. When I saw the table where the four of us had set so many times was set for three it was like going to our house the first time when Helen was not there. Jim and Ann were in the kitchen, so I went to the other room to get over the tears. I got to the "home" about 2:15. She was alone and in tears. She was always such a dignified lady. This just cannot be happening to her. I found it hard to talk with her about the good food when she was on the tube. When I left she reminded me Jim and Ann invited me to go back and pick up some turkey. She knows what is going on. There was no big change the next day.

The staff continues to tell me she is getting better. I can see that because she talks more than she did. However, she worries about not being able to get out of bed by herself. I can see how that would worry anyone. My big concern is she is not able to walk on her own. As of December 4th the big news is she is able to eat more like a normal meal.

I talked with the nurse manager December 5th about taking her out to dinner the next Tuesday night and then to the Christmas concert at our church. She said that would be good. Helen wanted to go, but was afraid of a kidney accident and said she had nothing to wear.

She ate practically all her dinner. The speech therapist is pleased with her progress. We discussed some personal things and she was alert. Her mind is working, but she continues to be depressed.

As of December 7th she was eating most of what they put on her tray, and they fed her less through the tube. We went out to eat with two other couples December 10th and then to the Christmas concert at out church. There were no problems and it was great.

She continues to eat well and talk rationally. I suggested going out to get some things she needs and she was concerned about being able to try them on. They continue to feed her liquids through the tube. We went to our house December 13th, but she could not get up the steps from the garage. We went to a Christmas program at Second Baptist December 14th and she enjoyed it. I thought she would be tired the next morning, Sunday, and I suggested we go to the evening service. When I got there Sunday after church a nurse told me she was disappointed I did not take her. We went to the evening service at our church. We were out together four nights this week.

When I got there December 17th at noon she had eaten about everything on her tray. She stands better now, but must have help to walk. I went to a seminar December 18th. When I got back a nurse told me she was concerned about me because of storm warnings she had seen on TV. We drove around December 20th sightseeing. We went to our house but she was unable to get up the steps to go into the house. She walked about 140 feet on the walker December 21st with me holding her. She is so discouraged that she cannot walk without help.

Sunday we went to Sunday school and church and then to our house. She was unable to get up the steps so we went to the nursing home.

It is Christmas Eve. I helped her dress before we went out to dinner and to the Christmas Eve service.

Can this be Christmas day? We had reservations at a restaurant for 12:30. When we got there on time we found the reservations meant nothing. Everyone stood in line. Most restaurants were closed. After a very good meal we took another drive and then went back to the nursing home.

Dec. 26th. I took her to the bathroom and she stood by the sink on her own for several minutes. I was close, but not touching her. We talked very seriously and I told her about the doctor saying November 3rd she would die in four to six weeks, and I said she is improving. She was concerned about not having anything to wear Saturday to our 40th anniversary dinner. She went to the closet, but could find nothing she had not worn two or three times.

After much talk it finally came—our 40th anniversary. We never dreamed it would be "celebrated" as a nursing home patient. Considering everything it was a very nice evening. She continues to be able to stand some on her own.

She seemed low December 30th. I believe that was because they had given her a shower and there is no privacy. After therapy I got her on the walker and she walked about 100 feet. We went to the New Year's Eve program at the church December 31st.

January 1ST 2O03 I took in a board game we enjoyed prior to her illness. She had forgotten a lot about it and was not too excited even though she played a fairly good game.

We took laundry home January 4th and a neighbor helped get her up the steps into the house. We had between three and four wonderful hours in our home together. Then out to eat and back to the nursing home.

January 6th I told her where I needed to go and asked if she wanted to go with me. She did not reply. Five or ten minutes later I told her I was going. Her actions, not her words, told me she wanted to go.

Wednesday, January 8th, we took some laundry home and were able to get her up the steps into the house. After doing the laundry we went to church. We were able to get up the steps again after the service. I got there shortly after lunch January 9th and she reminded me we did not get the clothes we took to the cleaners. January 11th we planned to heat a pizza at out home for lunch. We found the oven of our 28 year old stove was out so we ate out. We had about five hours together at our home.

Sunday, January 12th, we went to Sunday school and church, out to eat, and then home. It seemed more difficult to get her around on the walker.

We continue to talk about the time when she will go home to stay. I believe she will—at least I want to think she will. The doubt continues to haunt me. Will she ever go home to live? At my suggestion she called her old friend Ruth. She was alert, but weaker, January 15th.

When I got there the next day the first thing was to change her. Then I got her on the walker and she walked about 120 feet. She went to bed about 3:00 and slept about an hour.

When I got there January 18th I said something about going home the remainder of the day. She said nothing. When I took her to the bathroom she said something about what we should do before we leave. We went home. January 19th we went to church, out to eat, and then to another meeting I wanted to attend. When we got home she was so tired we did not attend the evening service. We went to the KFC to eat. She did not seem to know what to order. I finally ordered something light and she said she wanted the same. When the order came out she said she thought we were getting a full meal. I told her that before she got sick it was our custom to eat heavy Sunday at noon, as we did today, and light after church. I asked if she wanted more and she said no. She says so often she eats too much. This is typical of so many times she is not thinking normally. She says so often she wonders what is happening to her mind, or something to that effect. I try to tell her she is improving and to some extent I believe she is. What can I do? I try to be patient, but there are times———-.

When I got there about 1:15 January 20th she was in the wheel chair and appeared to have been there all day. I got her to bed about 2:20 and she slept about two hours. When she got up she said she did not want to eat at the nursing home. I took her to the bath room and then got her coat. She said she did not want to eat out. I reminded her of what she said before. We ate out, and she did not protest. After the study at church she thought I was getting in the wrong car. I showed her something in the back that convinced her. On the way to the nursissng home I tool the road we always take and she asked why we were going that way. She has always been better than me at reading maps on trips. I believe she is improving in many ways but recently I have noticed many things like I just mentioned. That concerns me.

After getting back to the nursing home we discussed, agreeably, the fact she does not like to go to bed so early. She has always been what I call a night owl. We agreed it is better for her to go to bed earlier so I can get to our house at a reasonable hour. She expressed her dissatisfaction with anyone else getting her ready for bed. The big news January 27th was I was told they would take out the feeding tube Friday and they did it.

She continues to be so silent, but she does talk some. I commented about that, and she said there is nothing to talk about. I said I can see her point but we must not give up, and we agreed on that. This is much easier said than done. Sunday, February 2nd, we had a chilli lunch for two

Sunday school classes after church. Many people paid special attention to her. After the lunch we went home for the afternoon.

February 4th I reminded her it was discount day at the Panda. She made no comment. About meal time I pushed her toward the dining room. She asked where her coat was. That told me she wanted to go to the Panda, and we went there for dinner. I believe she is so depressed about what she can do in the future that she believes, as she has said, there is nothing to talk about. We do talk some about the hope we have in our Lord—that He continues to be faithful. This is so discouraging to both of us. We talk about the possibility she will go home to live again. I want to believe she will go home, but still have that question. She very likely has the same question.

We went to the church dinner and prayer meeting February 19th. Betty Jo called me February 20 and said she was bringing over a chicken dinner for two. I took Helen home for that. It was wonderful for the two of us to eat at home together again. I should have learned to cook years ago. When we got back to the nursing home she was so tired and so sad. The next day she was in better spirits.

I got there about 3:45 February 22nd and she said this is the night for the couples club dinner. I had not planned to go because I thought it might be too much for her. We went.

It was snowing when I left February 24th. I got home safely and called her when I got home. I was snowbound the next two days, but called her each day. Thursday morning, the third day, I was able to get to my office. I saw her in the afternoon. When I left about 7:00 she gave me a big smile.

We ate out February 28th. I left a tip on the table and she asked what that was for. That is not like her because she was always so consicious of leaving a proper tip. We spent about an hour at our home.

Sunday, March 2nd, we went home for the afternoon. I brought out apple pie and ice cream in the mid afternoon. She said that was too much, but she ate her part and seemed to enjoy it.

We ate in the dining room March 3rd and then her actions, not her words, told me she wanted to go to the front area. It was a nice spring day, and we sat outside a half hour or so before subdown.

She spoke a few words to me when I got there March 4th. I suggested going to the front of the building so we could see outside. Much to my surprise she was willing to go. I asked where she wanted to eat and she did not say. I decided to go to the IHOP. She reminded me I had passed the Panda so I turned around and went back.

When I went in March 6th she had a smile on her face. I could take more of them. When I got there March 7th I suggested going home shortly after lunch tomorrow. That will be her 86th birthday. She gave me no answer, but I know she will like it. I picked her up about 2:00. In the mid afternoon we had pie and ice cream sitting at the table where we have enjoyed so many good meals. Do you say that is no big deal? Just wait till you and your spouse are parted for medical reasons and see.

We talked about the possibility of her coming home to live in April or May. We went home after church March 9th and she was very tired. Her getting so tired causes me to wonder how much I should take her out. And then there is the question of how much time she should spend in what I call "that place".

When I got there March 11th we visited Lucille, a patient. Helen joined in the conversation more than I have seen her do in a long time. She had a more satisfied look on her face. About 7:25 I suggested going back to her room because I needed to leave. She began to look sad. Every night is the same. I tell her how much I would like for us to spend the night together. She listens very closely, but says very little.

March 12th. Several people at the church commented on how much better she looks. That sounds good and she does look better. She cried when I left.

She puts up a good front and I admire her for that. When we are alone she falls apart. We spent Sunday afternoon at our house, and she was so tired she stayed in bed from 1:30 to 4:30.

Just before I left March 22nd I went over a number of the things we have done together. She said very little, but her expression showed she was interested and she agreed.

When I got there Sunday, March 23rd, she was the only patient in the dining room. She had a big breakfast on her tray, but had eaten very little except cereal. I took her to her room to dress . After church and eating out we went home. She started crying. I told her very firmly crying does no good and only disturbs both of us. I said if she cries all afternoon like she did last week I see no reason to come home. She cried very little after that. After the evening service we had a nice visit with friends at the K F C.

When we got to the "home" Wednesday night she was crying. All around it has not been a good day. People tell me this is harder on the caregiver (like me) than the patient (like her). I do not know how you can measure it. I do know it is stressful on both.

When I got there March 27th I told her friends from out of town are in the village and invited us to have dinner with them tomorrow. About 5:00 she asked when we were to meet them. I told her it was tomorrow, not today. We met them for dinner and a visit the next day, and then went to our home. I told her I would like her opinion on an idea I had. I said I hoped to have her home about three times a week after tax season when I have more time. I said it would take some time to move the office to our home, and we could come home Sunday afternoons as we do now, Wednesday afternoons, and some other time. I said we could see how that works out and then see if it was possible to bring her home for good. She said nothing. Then back to the nursing home where a friendly nurse met us. She asked if we had a good time. As a joke I said we had a rough time. I said we met two couples who were old friends, had dinner with them, and then went to our home. She got the point and made some choice remarks of her own. Helen laughed real good two or three times. It was the most I had heard her laugh in a long time.

When we got to church Sunday they had reserved a special seat for me where we could put her wheel chair in front of a pillar without blocking the isle and I could sit by her. When I got there Thursday she said something about where we were to go. Then she remembered the Easter program is tonight. I had planned not to go because she gets tired so easy. We went.

We went to the Good Friday service and then home. When we got up the steps at home she indicated, but did not say, she wanted to walk to her chair instead of using her wheel chair. We went to bed and I got up before she did. When I went back I found she had gotten up by herself and was walking toward the bathroom. It was good I got there when I did because she was getting very weak.

Her doctor said she is doing good but he had two concerns. One is her knee which he said can only be helped by a replacement. The other is her loss of weight. He said, and I agree, institutional food is institutional food. I told him I take her out to eat often and she eats good then. We went out to eat and she insisted on ordering only one side when two come with the dinner. I insisted on her ordering two and she finally did. She ate both. It is so sad to see her have such problems with such a minor thing when she was always such a brilliant lady.

When we got to the nursing home the next day I told her, as I have before, I believe she was hurt very bad before her first breakdown at age 24. She said she could not remember anything like that. I said I have heard of hurts that people drive back so far they cannot even remember them, but they come back later in different ways. I told her I knew one case very well where a man came back from World War ll wounded and later died. I said I met the lady he was engaged to and told her some of the things she told me. She said "you never told me that". I said I told her about the woman, but not so much detail. I told her I consider myself the winner because I have spent 40 years with her.

When I got there Sunday she had a big breakfast on her tray, but had eaten very little of it. I encouraged her to eat and spoon fed her some. She had lost at least twenty pounds since she got sick. After eating the noon meal she talked more than she did during the meal.

When I got there April 29th she needed a change. She started crying when we got in the bath room. I told her very firmly I could not continue to listen to her cry. It must have done some good because the crying decreased but did not stop. Then both of us slept some.

The next day we went home and I worked in the yard some. After about 20 minutes I went back and found her sleeping in the chair. When we went out to eat the next day she ate good and talked a little more.

We went home for lunch May 3rd. Betty Jo had given us some beef stew which made a delicious lunch. Going back to the nursing home brought the usual problems. When I left about 10:00 PM I went back to the empty house.

When I got there May 5th she was in fairly good shape. I asked if she wanted to eat out and she said she had two meals there today. We ate out.

We went out May 8th and I suggested getting her a new dress and pajamas. She said she did not know where to get them. That is not like her because she always knew where the best buys were. We went to Wal-Mart and she was at a total loss to know what to get. I chose a night gown that was too small.

We took a drive in the scenic mountains May 9th. After a short drive she told me we had been over that part before today. I did not say it but I thought it was dementia. Then I saw she was right and I was wrong. I told her she was right and I had made a wrong turn. We stopped at some scenic overlooks and she seemed to enjoy it. When we got back near the nursing home she started to sob.

When I got there about 1:30 May 10th she was in the wheel chair and was very tired. She had probably been in the chair all day. I know the staff has a lot to do but it seems she gets so tired after being in the chair too long. I took her to the bathroom and then we laid down for over an hour. She was more relaxed then. We went to visit friends and then to our home. I started the next day doing some very serious thinking. I know she has serious problems. This leads to serious problems for me and I have taken mine too seriously. Really, I have been selfish in expecting too much from her. The next day was not a good day and I lost all my good intentions.

Sunday when we got to our house she walked on the walker and was not in the wheel chair. When we got to the church for the evening service I told her she would use the walker and not the chair. I did the same when we went out to eat. She talked with me at the restaurant, and talked some on the way to the nursing home.

It may sound like I am cruel. I hate to do some of the things I have done. I have told her I have feelings too. I try to help her in every way I can. I asked her what she would do if I died first and she did not reply.

When I got there the next day she talked with me as soon as I walked in. We lay on the bed a while and when she woke she talked some with me.

We went to Wal-Mart to get her some clothes, and she was able to pick out what she wanted. She was more like the lady I was married to long ago. She did take more time, but she knew what she liked. I saw a seat and went to it and sat where I could watch her.

She was in better spirits and talked more May 13th. When we got home about 4:30 she walked by herself on the walker a big part of the way across the living room to her chair.

When I got there about 11:00 she was in bed and had her pajamas on. A nurse told me she refused to get up and they took her breakfast to her and she ate in bed. I got her up and dressed her, but she would not talk. We ate lunch out and went home. About 5:30 I mentioned going out for a drive and she did not reply. A few minutes later she started moving around in her chair. This told me she was ready to go. She did not say yes or no. I intentionally let her go a few minutes before helping her. We went for a drive and then out to eat.

When I got there Sunday, May 18th, she was in bed and the nurse told me she refused to get up. I just started getting her up. Her breakfast was brought to the room while we were in the bathroom. She ate a little without my encouragement and then at my insistence she ate a reasonable breakfast. I chose what she wore and a nurse dressed her.

When I got there May 19th she appeared to be in fair shape. I took her downtown because I needed to deliver some papers and then we went home. I asked her to look over some things I plan to put in a garage sale. I did this with some reservations because I thought it might be too much for her. She said she would be ashamed for anyone to see the room because it was in such a mess. We discussed how we would arrange things after I move certain things from my office. I was working with my back to her and since she was in the wheel chair I saw no need to watch her closely. I turned and, to my amazement, she had gotten up by herself and was standing on her feet. We worked on the project thirty or forty minutes. Now I believe it was a challenge to her mind. She seemed more like the lady I married. When I left the nursing home about 10:00 she was in bed and not crying.

We went to our home a little over an hour after church May 21st. When we left she seemed to hesitate more and more. I have no doubt it was because she did not want to leave home, and she knew where she was going. When we got to the nursing home she was crying more than she has in several days.

She asked me May 23rd what I had done about moving the office.

When we went home May 24th she was in bed from about 1:30 till 4:00. Then she walked on her walker past the chair where she usually sits. She walked to the kitchen and just stood there ten or fifteen minutes. She must have been thinking about the time she has spent there since we moved here almost eighteen years ago, and wondering if she would ever prepare another meal for the two of us.

The next day, Sunday, when I got there she was in the dining room, but had eaten practically nothing. I spoon fed her two or three bites of scrambled eggs and bacon. Then she started eating and ate a fair amount. I took her to her room and dressed her for church.

I have talked with her about what to expect when she gets home. Really, I am not sure what to expect, but I want her back as soon as possible.

When we got home May 26th I showed her what I had done in her studio room to make it possible to move some of my office equipment there. She sat in a regular chair, looked the place over, and made several suggestions which I appreciated. We sat in that room about half an hour. She seemed more like the lady I married and have lived with a little over forty years. I mentioned eating watermellon and she acted like that was too much. I cut somme for both of us and she seemed to enjoy it. We went out to eat about 6:30. I ordered a regular meal and she would not order anything but a sandwich. After ordering she said she may have made a mistake. I tried to get her to change her order, but she would not. Then we went home and ate ice cream. She said she felt like she was stuffed. I said I do not want her to starve. We talked a lot about her coming home soon. When I left her at the nursing home she was in tears.

Her voice sounds so much better today. Prior to her illness her voice was normally loud and clear. For a long time it has been so low I can hardly hear her a lot of the time. Today I could understand her very clearly. At the restaurant she complained, as usual, about them bringing out too much food, but she ate most of her fish dinner. When I left her at the nursing home she was not crying.

She talked to me when I got there May 28th. We went by the house and got the mail before going to church. We went to our house after church. I hope to have her back to live at home in two or three weeks. I do not know what to expect when she gets home. It is really scary to think what her reaction would be if something happened that she could not come home to live.

We have had a few very good days recently. Today, May 29th, was not one of them.

When I got there about 4:00 May 30th I found her in bed asleep and in her night clothes. I asked an LPN what she knew about her and she said "nothing". I could see she was busy, but it was also obvious she did not care. I went to the director of nursing. Later a young black lady asked me about Helen. It was obvious she did care. The LPN mentioned above said that was the day shift's job. I took her to the village to eat dinner and then we went home.

I prepared a ham sandwich for lunch at home May 31st. When I brought out watermellon she said that was too much. We sat on the back porch awhile and then I worked in the yard. I could see her most of the time.

When I got there Sunday, June 1st, she was in the dining room and her tray was almost empty. From what I have seen before she must have eaten a good breakfast. Her mood was not good. After church we had dinner with Wayne and Ruth again. Then we had a good afternoon at home.

She talked with me quite a bit June 2nd. At home we went to the room where I plan to put the computer. She stood without my help or a walker and really looked things over in a professional way. She made several good suggestions. She was more like the Helen of years ago, and I told her that. I really believe she will come home soon.

When we are away from the nursing home I encourage her to use the walker or walk with me holding her. Several times she has walked on her own from the bathroom. This may be dangerous, but I have not discouraged it. Sometimes I walk away when she is at the sink. This may help her build confidence.

We went out for lunch June 7th and then home. I insisted on playing UpWords and she said it was the dumbest game she ever saw. At my insistence we went to Alco and purchased some things for her.

When I got there Sunday she was in the dining room dressed for church and it appeared she had eaten a good breakfast. I showed her a letter I had written to the director of nursing saying I plan to take her home not later than June 21st. She agreed with it, but had practically nothing to say.

The next day at home I turned my back on her while she was on the walker. When I looked back she was at least ten feet from her walker.

We came home after church June 15th and sat on the back porch awhile. I went in the house for something. When I went back she had gotten up, opened the door, and gone to her usual chair withour my help.

Two things really stand out with me from her experience in the nursing home. One is that so many people are taken there and seem to be forgotten, or just dumped there. They have very few, if any, visitors. The other is I visited Helen every day except two days I was snowed in. I tried to take her out as often as possible. I believe that encouraged her, and was the reason for a big part of her recovery.

SHE COMES HOME TO LIVE

She came home to live June 16, 2003. That was six days short of ten months away from home. She walked from her chair to her studio and started talking about how she would ever get her studio cleaned up. I told her such worrying would send her back to the hospital and I would not permit that. When we woke the next morning she asked if we had anything in the house for breakfast. We did and we had breakfast about like what we enjoyed before her illness. She has always liked to stay up late, so we watched the 700 Club on TV till it ended at 11:00 PM. We enjoyed that program before her illness. We went to the grocery store and she used the grocery cart as a "walker". She seemed to sleep good the first two nights, and recovery is coming along better than I expected.

The third day we took a trip of about twenty miles to get something for my computer. I think we probably overdid it because she was very tired at the end of the day.

Shortly after she got sick the oven on our twenty-eight year old stove went out. Ruth, who has helped so much, went downtown with us to help Helen choose some clothes. After Helen and I agreed on a stove they went to the ladies' department while I closed the deal on the stove.

She did not sleep good the night of June 20-21. I noticed she had not taken her medicine the night before. She did not want to take her medicine after breakfast. Ruth came back to help her try on her new dress. I went out about 3:00 to mow the lawn. She did not talk with me the first two times I came in to check on her. After dinner she did not want to take her medicine.

She was so silent Sunday, June 22nd. After the evening service she told me she had a spot on the new dress she was wearing for the first time. The next day I made an appointment with her doctor and was told she had shingles. She had this when she left the nursing home, but it had not been diagnosed as such. The next morning she dressed with very little help from me and walked to the kitchen without the walker or help from me. Then at 11:30 she walked to the bathroom without my help. Two electricians came at 1:30 to do some work putting in the new range. She brought up a good point I had not thought about. When they left she was very tired.

We were awake at 3:30 AM June 25th and she seemed OK. When we woke again at 6:30 she was crying. I asked if she took her medicine last night and she said no. I had watched her take her potassium and medicine for the shingles, but had not watched for the other. I had to dress her. When she first came home one of my major concerns was she might have trouble with kidney control. This has not been a problem. She is now able to get to the bathroom without help. She seemed better when she woke June 26th, and did not need help dressing. I needed to go out at 3:15 and took her with me. She was very tired when we got back, and at bed time. She was not able to dress herself the next day. About noon I found a pachage on the porch the UPS had left. She said I got one like that yesterday. Oh that dementia.

I turned on the TV a little after 10:00 to get the 700 Club, a program we enjoyed before her illness. She started crying about 10:45 and that told me she was too tired to continue watching it. It was not nice of me, but I told her she should tell me in words, and not cry.

When we woke the next morning I helped her put on her underclothes and then I walked out. She finished dressisng. I asked twice what she wanted for breakfast, and she did not tell me. When we went downtown for dinner she talked a little while we ate.

June 29th has been one of her best days recently. She used her walker to walk from the Sunday school room to the sanctuary which is quite a distance. She had a better expression on her face in mid afternoon. I suggested she read a letter from Dr James Dobson which I had just read. She read it and said enough to tell me she appreciated it.

We have a fellowship tonight after the church service. People take food but it is not a regular dinner. In mid afternoon she remembered that and made a good suggestion about what we should take.

When we woke June 30th she said she probably slept some. She whimpered some after she got to the bathroom. She began the usual about not having anything to put on. I said she had clothes in the closet as I walked out. All around it was a good morning. She talked some at lunch. About 10:30 PM it was obvious she was tired and needed to go to bed.

She was in a bad mood when we woke July 1st, and I had to help her dress. She has not wanted to take her medicine lately and I let her get away with that last night. She is so quiet. I wonder how much good the medicine does, but I am afraid to let her stop taking it. At 9:00 PM she was very tired and I helped her get ready for bed.

She dressed herself July 2nd, but it took a long time. She sat in her chair most of the morning except for the time we sat on the back porch. After lunch we took the lawn mower to the shop, and then went to the grocery store. She used the grocery cart as a walker.

When we woke July 4th she seemed to be in fair shape. I went to the kitchen and then back after about 20 minutes. I dressed her and then she walked to the kitchen by herself. After lunch we drove up Scenic 7 and after about 10 miles she said go back home. I asked where she wanted to eat dinner and she gave me no answer. As we drove by KFC she said she wanted to eat there. I drove back and she was very quiet. When we got home she was so tired I insisted she go to bed and she slept about an hour.

She was not able to dress herself Sunday. She purchased a new dress about two weeks ago and I asked if she wanted to wear it. She did not seem to remember it. That is not like her. She used the walker today. I tell her she should use it as it helps exercise her legs. I was up about 4:00 AM and I am not sure she knew when I got up or went back to bed. That is not like her, as she was always a very light sleeper and knew when I got up or went back to bed.

I have spent a lot of time typing this the last ten months. What will I ever do with it? I really do not know. Will I ever show it to her? Again, I do not know.

When she got out of bed the next day I had to do a big part of dressing her. I was very careful to see she took her medicine. She did not want to take it. I am afraid for her not to take it, but I wonder if she could be weaned away from it a little at a time. After breakfast she walked past her chair to the bedroom. As I was making the bed she stopped at the door of the bedroom and just looked around. This is July 8th 2003 and we have lived here almost eighteen years. We talked about some important and personal things. She went on a 3 ½ mile trip with me to see a client. After dinner as a joke I asked her to get on her stationery bike for a ride.

She looked at it seriously. Then I got serious. She got on the bike and turned the pedal ten times.

The next day Joe and Carolyn brought over some delicious food for lunch. We went downtown and then had dinner at home. While I was preparing dinner she walked across the room to the dining table without her walker. She was very tired when she went to bed.

She dressed without my help July 10th. About 3:30 PM I found her crying in her chair and found it was bedcause she needed to go to the bathroom.

July 12th started off better than the last few days. I helped her start dressing and then walked out. Later in the day I noticed she did not put on hose. We went to the grocery in the afternoon. After dinner I suggested a game of UpWords and told her that would make her think. She agreed but with reservations. She played a fair game at the beginning, but was very tired when we finished. The next day she was very quiet. I needed to go out so we ate lunch out. As she was preparing for bed she said, as she has said many times, "I can't go out there like this." I told her, as I have before, there was no one here but us. When she got to the shower she had a blouse on.

Ruth came over July 16th and did some cooking for us. After Ruth left I told Helen I did not know where the carrying case was that she used to carry hot dishes. She said it was in the closet and she found it immediately. She had not seen it since before her illness almost a year ago. About 9:00 PM it was obvious she was tired. I asked if she wanted to go to bed and she said she did.

She went with me to see my eye doctor and heard everything the doctor said. She was concerned when the doctor said the stroke I had almost four years ago affected my brain. Near bed time she seemed to be better than she has been at bed time in several days.

She reminded me July 18th that we should pick up some things I had forgotten. In mid-afternoon, with very little encouragement from me, she rode her stationery bike. She turned the pedals twenty times, or twice what she did July 8th. She went with me to the grocery July 19th. I was very discouraged because she would not, or could not, talk with me. It was not nice of me, but I told her she could talk with me, get out of the chair on her own, or just sit there. After about twenty minutes she got on her feet by herself. About 4:00 PM she rode the bike a little further than she did yesterday. I keep telling her not to give up. She was so tired she went to bed about 9:00 PM.

The next day she turned the pedals on the bike 35 times. She stayed up till 10:00 PM. She was very tired. I raised the question of how much good the medicine is doing. She said it is not helping the problem, but it is causing the problem. I believe she could be right. I am afraid of what so much medicine is doing to her, but I am afraid for her to stop it. What can I do?

She frequently cries when she gets out of bed in the morning. Very frequently I help her start dressing and then walk out just to see if she can dress herself. Sometimes it works and sometimes I go back and dress her.

We went to bed a little before 10:00 July 22nd and she seemed a little sad at first. I have no idea why she did it or why it seemed funny. As we lay there she held my chin and looked in my mouth. She started laughing and said it looked dark in there. I told her I had not heard her laugh that much in months. I did not even suggest she take any medicine the next morning.

Alzheimer's, Depression and Dementia

Ruth came the next day to do some cooking for us. Then Ruth went to the store for us and said everything on the stove would be OK till she got back. I went to the living room about 11:50 to check on Helen. She had gotten out of the chair without help and walked to the stove and back to the hall, or a distance of about 50 feet. She said she wondered about what was on the stove. I asked if she thought we should take the wheel chair back to the loan closet where we borrowed it. She said very little. I parked near the door and she pushed the chair inside.

I warmed up the dinner Ruth cooked. At the table I mentioned several of the interesting things we had done during our marriage. I asked her to name some of the things that stood out in her mind during our long marriage. She waited three or four minutes before answering. Imagine my thrill when she mentioned our honeymoon. What man could ask for anything more? After dinner she was very low again. I helped her get out of the chair and on her feet. I said it was good for her to be on her feet more and in the chair less. She did not talk much, but seemed to agree with what I said.

When we woke the next morning she talked in such a clear voice it was much like it was years ago. I complimented her on that. She would not take her medicine and I did not insist on her doing it. After breakfast she walked to the back porch and to the bike. Then she said no. I laughed at her and then she got on it and turned the pedals 72 times. When I got ready to warm up dinner she indicated she wanted to go to the kitchen and I gladly helped her walk to the kitchen. I got something from the frig and then she stopped in front of the frig door. I asked her to move so I could open the frig door again. She moved and started crying. I told her if she was going to cry to get out of the kitchen because I could not work with her crying. The meal Ruth cooked was good, but the atmosphere was bad. We watched a TV program we liked before her illness. At 9:00 PM it was obvious she was very tired so I helped her go to bed. When we woke the next morning she was more alert and talked normally quite a bit. I had to help dress her. She walked to the kitchen without the walker. After eating she walked to the back porch . With considerable insistance from me she did the bike ride. I had a 9:30 appointment. At 8:30 she said it was time to go. It was only a five minute drive, but that showed she was thinking.

The next day did not start off well as she did not talk. I helped her start dressing and then walked out to see what she would do. About mid morning she went to the bike and did 90 turns. Then she indicated she wanted to go to the kitchen and I walked there with her. She seemed to want to look things over and, I am sure, was thinking of all the things she had done there.

Since she has not been able to work in the kitchen she has a lot to learn about the new range and microwave. It seems so strange for me to show her anything about the kitchen. She was always such a wonderful cook. She took the place mats off the top of the frig and put them on the table. This sounds so simple, but for so long she was not able to take one step by herself. Prior to preparing dinner I had really unloaded my heart to her by telling her many things that happened while she was in the hospital and nursing home. One doctor had told me he expected her to die more than seven months ago. We went to bed about 10:00 PM and had a normal conversation till about 11:30. What a wonderful time.

I asked what she wanted for lunch and she said we had nothing to prepare. We had plenty, but I took that to mean she wanted to go out. We ate out. About 7:00 PM I suggested she call her old friend Ruth. While they were talking I wrote a letter to an old friend of hers who wrote us about six months ago. Just as I finished she walked into the room where I was at the computer. I asked her to write whatever she wanted to. It took her an hour to type two sentencesd on the computer.

We got up about 7:15 the next morning and I went to the computer. Then I went to the kitchen and found her there preparing cereal. That was great and I told her so. After church we went out to eat and then to a board meeting at Potter's Clay. She walked quite a bit without help. When we got home she rode the bike about 3/10 of a mile. She has walked more today than I can remember since she got sick. When we woke July 28th she was talking normally. Then when she got up things went bad. I did not offer to help her dress because I wanted to see what she could do.

We had an appointment with her regular physician July 29th. The doctor seemed to be surprised at how much improvement she had made. He asked if she needed any refills on the prescriptions he had given her. He told her to keep on doing what she had been doing. I did not tell him that since a week ago yesterday she had taken only two pills and that was a week ago tonight.

She continues to show improvement, but also continues to be so depressed. She walks more on her own and does more on the stationery bike. That thrills me. I know our Lord has not promised us we would live here forever, but when should you give up and not want to live any more, or the same for someone you love? She got up without help July 31st, walked to the bathroom, and back to bed. I did very little to help dress her. She did 100 turns on the stationery bike. A lady at our church told me Helen's case sounds very similar to her mother's. August 2nd we made two short walks of about 75 feet "round trip" each in front of our house. I woke at 1:00 AM August 3rd and found her crying. The same thing about an hour later. We got up about 7:00. I walked out and told her to dress herself. I have learned she can do what she wants to do even though it takes a long time to do it. I told her she is going back on her regular medicine till she gets better. She took it, but did not want to. I should have been more polite. She did her bike ride and then we sat on the back porch about half an hour.

When she got up the next morning the first thing she said was something about not having anything to wear. She has plenty clothes.

I suggested two places we could go for dinner and she did not reply. When I drove past the first place she said she thought we were goine there. I went back. I said she can talk when she wants to. That was not nice of me. She looked very tired about 9:00 PM and I asked if she wanted to go to bed. She said no. A few minutes lated I could tell she needed to go to bed and I asked her again. She did not reply. I told her when she told me she was ready I would help her, and till then she could sit in her chair. About fifteen minutes later she squirmed in her chair. When she finally said she was ready I helped her get up and go to bed.

We have a Billy Graham video which I saw before she got sick. She said she did not remember seeing it. I believe we saw it together, but she forgot it. I put it on and it was so much like her illness we took it off and watched a musical video. We slept very little that night. She got to the kitchen before I did the next morning, and I found her standing by the stove. She fried the eggs and watched as I put the sausage in the microwave. I consider this a definite improvement.

The next day the Smiths, missionary friends of ours, came about 5:00 PM. We went out to eat and then stayed up later than usual. She was very tired when we went to bed. Catherine enjoyed cooking breakfast and I was thrilled for her to do it. We went to church where Ralph told of their work with Wycliffe. She was up later than she should have been. We enjoyed having our friends visit, but it was too much for her. Her crying woke me at 2:10 AM and again at 5:15. She watched very closely when Ralph showed me some things on the computer.

Shortly after we ate lunch it was time to empty the clothes dryer. She took some things out of the dryer and I did not tell her she should or should not do that. She folded the sheets and we went to the bedroom where the visitors had slept. They had made the bed with sheets from the closet. She wanted to use the sheets we used on that bed before she got sick, so we changed the linens. It was good to see she was thinking. And she was talking. What a change in less than an hour. When we went out to eat she said they brought out too much food, but she ate most of it.

She was so tired August 12th I insisted she go to bed at 8:00 PM. I said she night want to get up and see the 700 Club. She got up at 9:45 and went back to bed at 10:30.

We woke at 5:15 AM Aug. 13th and she said she had to get up. I asked why and she did not reply. She got up about 8:00. She did her bike ride and walk on the back porch. We went downtown about 10:30 to get some work done on the car air conditioner. We had lunch downtown and she was so tired when we got home. It amazes me how little it takes to make her so tired. There is always that question of whether it is better to take her when she gets tired so easy, or get someone to stay with her at home where she would get cabin fever. I have chosed to take her with me when I can. About bed time I remembered I had not given her the potassium. She cried, but she took it. I told her I would come to bed when she quit crying.

I dressed her the next morning and told her to sit in her chair till I got breakfast. I told her I cannot work when she is standing near me crying. After breakfast she did 110 turns on the bike. She talked a little at lunch. We went downtown and stopped at the bank. I showed her a check I was cashing for $100.00 and she seemed surprised.

I helped her start dressing Aug. 15th and then walked out. When I went back she was almost dressed. The next day was almost repeat. When I started getting dinner she asked in a crying voice what I was doing. Sunday, Aug. 17th, started off bad. I heard her crying about 6:00 AM. I knew that meant she needed to go to the bathroom. The only word she spoke was when I asked if she got a good night's sleep. Later she said she did not have anything to wear. I hear that so often. Dressing her was more difficult than usual. As she walked toward the kitchen I told her to sit in the chair till I got breakfast ready.

Monday morning she did her bike ride and then walked the length of the porch and back. When I suggested she take the second walk on the porch she said she thought she had done it twice. Oh, that dementia. The next morning she dressed herself even though it took a long time for her to do it.

New people have purchased the house next door. They have remodeled it. They invited us to see it and we did that today. She always loved things like that before she got sick. I believe she enjoyed it, but she said very little.

Alzheimer's, Depression and Dementia

What is it like to see something you have always enjoyed, and know you are not able to enter into that now? It must be sad.

She did most of dressing herself Aug. 20th. About 9:00 PM I asked if she wanted to go to bed. She said no. About ten minutes later I could see she was very tired, and I told her it was time to go to bed. She was almost in tears. I got her to bed about 9:30 and told her I would join her when she quit crying. I went to bed about 11:00 and she was rather calm.

When she woke Aug. 21st she talked in a very clear voice. I was on Cloud 9. When she came back from the bathroom the talk was over. I had to help her dress and it was a job. When I started to warm up Ruth's cooking for dinner Helen thought I was putting too much on the plates. After eating breakfast I suggested walking out front. Then I suggested walking down our drive which is very steep. When we walked back I saw that walking down and up that steep drive is very dangerous for her. I was scared as we walked back up the drive, and I decided not to do that again till she gets better.

Today's mail included a letter from a Wycliffe couple who spent the night with us a couple of years ago. After reading it I showed it to her. I am sure she was interested, but she said very little.

I worked in the yard some and she thought I was doing too much. We had a dinner party with the Couple's Club at 6:00 and at 3:30 she said she did not know what to do. I asked what she meant and she said about getting ready. I got her ready. She seemed to enjoy the meeting but said very little to the three couples who were at the table with us.

She was crying when she got to the kitchen the next morning. I took her back to the chair and told her I would get her when breakfast was ready. She ate a good breakfast. We heard there were to be some very interesting lights in the sky tonight so she stayed up later to see them. We went to the back porch at 9:30 and stayed there till after 10:00, but saw no lights. She was very tired when I helped her to bed.

We woke about 7:00 Aug. 25th and she started the old routine about having nothing to wear. I told her she had clothes and she can buy more when she feels like going out and choosing what she wants. She got up about 7:45 and seemed to be at a total loss about what to put on, or what to let me put on her. I prepared breakfast and just as I started back to tell her breakfast was ready I saw her coming to the kitchen. Breakfast went quite well and she did the back porch routine.

When it was about time to get lunch she was near the kitchen and she said she did not know what to do. I said "to do about what?" She said about what to fix for lunch. I told her I would be there soon and told her what we have to prepare. She said she wanted a fish sandwich. I told her what to do at the stove and commented on how strange it is for me to show her anything about the kitchen. The longer she stood there the more she sobbed. I rested a few minutes after lunch and then went to the office. Then I went back to the living room and found her standing in the middle of the room looking around as if she were deciding how to change the place. Or maybe she was thinking about something else—who knows? I went to the grocery alone. When I got back and was putting the groceries away I looked up and saw her standing nearby. She had gotten out of the chair without my help and was almost in tears. I told her I know she is hurting because she cannot do what she wants to do, but I notice she got out of the chair by herself and came to the kitchen to cry about what I was doing. That was not nice of me.

I got up about 2:30 AM and went to the bathroom. When I went back she was in her bathroom. I commented on her getting up by herself and she said "yeah, but I almost fell."

Aug. 27th started off not too different. Marie came in by appointment and started to tell me a story I thought Helen would enjoy. We went to the other room and found Helen taking the laundry out of the dryer. She talked a little more than usual tonight. About 9:00 I asked if she wanted to go to bed and she said no. Ten minutes later she was so tired she was ready for bed.

We woke about 7:00 the next morning and she said she had to get up. I asked why and she did not reply. That has happened before. I helped start dressing her and then walked out. Some time later she came to the kitchen fully dressed.

She was awake at 5:15 and said it was time to get up. I told her Sunday school starts at 9:30 or in about four hours. We got up at 7:20 and I had to dress her. We had lunch at home and a church picnic and dinner at 5:00.

She was crying when she woke Sept. 1st. I helped her start dressing and then I walked out. About twenty-five minutes later I went back. Since she had not dressed I finished dressing her. When I was preparing lunch she came to the kitchen crying. I took her back to the chair and told her to stay there till lunch was ready. We woke about 4:45 AM Sept. 2nd and she said it was time to get up. We got up about 7:00, and she was in tears. I walked out hoping she would dress herself, but she did not.

The next day she talked a little as she went to the bathroom. She said she needed to get some clothes on. I told her I agreed with that and she started crying. I left the room and I dressed. Then I went back about twenty minutes later and dressed her. I suggested going to the Panda for dinner since that was discount day, and she said nothing. When I said I was ready she was ready too. When we got in line at the buffet she acted like she did not know what to do. At my insistence she started putting food on her plate and she ate a good meal. On the way home I said she had an appointment with her hair dresser tomorrow at 2:00. Very quickly she said it was at 1:45. When we got home I checked my appointment book and found she was right.

She talked a very little when she got up the next day.

The afternoon of September 5th went quite well. When it was time to get dinner it appeared she wanted to go to the kitchen, but she was near tears. I helped her up, and told her she could go to the kitchen only if she did not cry. Then she sat down in her chair. I helped her up when dinner was ready.

When we woke September 7th she was near tears. I helped dress her. After breakfast I went to the utility room and when I came back she was standing near the stove. I said nothing. Later I saw she had the frig door open. I asked what she needed, and she said she just wanted to see what we had. I told her I liked that.

After the evening church service I left her in the pew and went to the front of the church to talk with the visiting speaker. She walked to the front where I was. She is improving in her ability to walk and today I noticed a definite improvement in her speech. This tells me she is improving.

The next day I helped her start dressing and then walked out. Just as I started eating she came to the kitchen properly dressed. She ate a normal breakfast and did it in a normal time. She frequently eats so slow it is cold before she finishes. Then she did the back porch routine. When it was time to get dinner it was obvious she wanted to go to the kitchen. She was almost in tears. I told her she could go to the kitchen, but only if she did not cry. I helped her up from the chair and went to the kitchen. She stood by the chair awhile and then sat down. I helped her to the table when dinner was ready. She was very sad when she went to bed. I tried to talk with her, but that did not go over very well.

She talked a little more September 9th.

I find that a big part of the time when she gets out of bed I can help her start dressing, and then walk out, and she can finish dressing even though it takes her a long time.

She was in the kitchen while I prepared dinner September 13th and did not cry. We had a quiet, but pleasant, dinner.

I did most of the dressing her September 14th but to some extennt that was because we got up late and I did not want to be late for church. The afternoon at home was so quiet. It is so sad to sit in the same room with someone you have lived with and loved for forty years and have no communications.

September 17th I took her to a ladies' breakfast that started at 8:45, and picked her up when it was over. On the way home I asked her about the program. She said a lady from Texas spoke. I asked what she talked about and she said she talked about her life. She said nothing more.

We woke about 5:00 AM and she was sobbing. I took her to the bathroom and the sobbing ceased. We went back to sleep till about 7:00. She said something about sleeping too late. She dressed much quicker than usual. Without hesitation she told me what she wanted for breakfast. We had a much better breakfast and then she did the back porch routine. We went downtown for lunch and then to the state park. Before we got to the park she asked how much father we were going. I told her I thought it was about ten miles further. She had a handicapped parking permit. When we got to the Lodge I saw a handicapped parking place and said "I am handicapped you know". She said "Yeah, you're handicapped because of me." I told her that was not true. I said we have had problems the last year or so, but we have had many years of blessings. We went inside and looked over the lake for half an hour or so and then home. She talked more, and more rationally, today than she has in a long time. When we got home I said we have had a good day. She said "We have" and then laughed out loud.

When we woke the next day she was not crying but she was not talking either. She did tell me what she wanted for breakfast. We walked some out front. She is not feeling as well as she did yesterday at the park. She talked more Sunday at church and Sunday school, and when we went out to eat she had less trouble ordering. When we got home she seemed to be more tired. Who can tell what to expect? She was so tired when she got to bed about 9:40 PM. She was much better Thursday and worse Friday. She was better Saturday and not so good today. I really wonder how much longer she will live. I know it is in the hands of our Lord. Both of us have lived long lives.

There was really nothing too different the next few days. Getting started in the morning continues to be a problem. September 25th she indicated she wanted to get out of the chair about 4:00 PM. I tell her she needs to spend more time on her feet and less time in the chair. We walked out on the walk and then sat on the front porch. She was in a better mood. I said nothing about her going to the kitchen as I was preparing dinner. Just before I finished I noticed she was getting nervous so I helped her out of the chair. Dinner went quite well and there was some talk. Any talk is an improvement.

We had plans to meet friends for dinner so I insisted she wear a dress and not slacks. She said we were to meet them at the restaurant at 5:00. We got there at 5:20 and were the second couple to arrive. After eating we went to the home of one of the couples for desert and a visit. The men went to one room and the ladies to another. When we got ready to leave and we got to the room where the ladies were I saw a smile on Helen's face like I had not seen in a long time. And the smile stayed there a long time compared to what I have seen recently. As we were going home she said I was going the wrong way even though I was going the right way, and she has always been the best navigator on trips. She was very tired and got to bed about 10:00. When I went to bed I slept till about 11:30 and could not go back to sleep. I got up about 12:00 and read about an hour. When I went back to bed she said she had not been asleep. We had a nice talk and she talked very rationally. This is only the second time we have had a normal talk in the three months since she came home from the nursing home. I told her how happy I was. When she woke in the morning she was sobbing and it was the old routine.

The next morning when she woke she was crying but that almost stopped when I took her to the bath room. I asked if she slept good and she said she thought she did. I put her underclothes on her and walked out as I told her to put on a dress. When I went back she had a dress on that was OK but she had no hose on and a pair of shoes she would not normally wear to church. I commented about that and she said she did not have any hose. I got hose and a better pair of shoes for her. Breakfast went OK.

We ate out after church with a couple we had not seen recently. Later at home she mentioned the party Friday night. I told her it was last night, not Friday night. She was wrong about the date, but she was talking. She also said something about her mind not working right. I told her that was true, but I could see definite signs of improvement. I was being honest with her. She also asked if it was this coming Wednesday, Thursday, and Friday I was to go to a seminar. I told her she was right.

There was a little small talk when we woke about 6:00 AM. When I took her to the bathroom she commented about the heat coming out of the register. She has talked so little for so many months any talk is a big thing for me. We went back to bed and her mood changed completely. She complained about the way I was cooking and I asked her to fry her own bacon. She did and I considered that an improvement. In the evening we had a friendly heart to heart talk. After that I held her close and asked the Lord to free both of us from whatever was binding us. Both of us seemed more released. Is released the proper word?

Breakfast was not too good the next day. When I was ready to get lunch I asked if she wanted to go to the kitchen. She did not reply so I left her in the chair. I got her when lunch was ready. Dinner went rather well even though there was very little talk. After dinner I popped some pop corn without telling her I was going to do it. She ate a fair amount. I started to refill her bowl and she covered her bowl with her hand, and said a definite no. I told her I would have to eat the rest of it. She told me not to do that. I ate some more, but not all of it.

I had a seminar the next three days, but was home each night and had someone with her all time I was gone. There was nothing else too different during those three days.

When she woke the next morning she seemed to be better, but not so good after she went to the bathroom. Abouit 4:00 PM I insisted she get out of her chair and move around some. I told her Dr Dobson wrote that love must be tough. There was no big difference the next day.

After church I talked with Bev who stayed with Helen when I was at the seminar. She said they talked some but Helen seemed to stare into space some of the time. While we were talking Helen walked up behind me and I told her Bev and I were talking about her.

Getting up the next day was about the old routine with me helping her start dressing, walking out, and waiting for her to dress. While I was preparing dinner she came to the kitchen and started crying. I took her to her chair and then got her back when dinner was ready. At first I thought her crying was being critical of my work. It is probably because she cannot do what she always loved and did so well. Whatever the reason it is difficult for me to work with her crying nearby.

A couple of days later she was not in a good mood when she woke but she dressed herself and was in the kitchen earlier than usual. The next day, October 9th, she did not know what to wear. I practically forced her to let me dress her and then walked out. She got to the kitchen while I was eating breakfast.

I was reading a book she did not recognize. She asked what it was and I told her it was a tax book I got at the seminar last week. It was good to hear her voice, but I only answered her question. Sometimes it is difficult to know how much I should say.

When I was preparing lunch she was sitting about twenty feet from where I was. In a crying voice she asked what I was fixing. I told her I was preparing lunch and I would get her when it was ready. This was another meal that was not pleasant, and I was the one who was crying.

The next day she said she did not know what to wear. I chose something and she said she would not wear that. We went to the grocery that morning. One time she acted like she was about to cry. I told her if she cried we would leave the store. I asked her to go to the kitchen to see what she wanted me to cook for dinner. She made no suggestion, but started crying. I took her by the arm and set her in the chair by the table till I got dinner. After eating I showed her a recipe Ruth had written for me which I had requested. I thought it was her recipe for chicken and rice which I love. She never made any comment.

Both of us went to the bathroom about 4:30 AM October 12th. When we got back to bed we had a pleasant conversation. That was great. When we got up about 7:00 it was a completely different story. When we went out to eat after church she had difficulty ordering, but not as much as I have seen.

Again, we woke about 4:00 AM October 14th and had a pleasant conversation.

She attended a ladies' breakfast October 15th and a lady friend brought her home. Lunch at home went OK. After eating a sandwich I mentioned three choices for desert. After I asked twice she did not respond. Then I asked if she said one of each. Then in the plainest and loudest language I had heard from her in a long time she said " I did not say one of each". I told her I like that understandable voice. We had a good conversation after we went to bed and I was on Cloud 9.

She had problems dressing October 16th and I finished dressing her. I asked what she wanted for breakfast and she did not tell me. When she got to the kitchen I suggested she prepare her own breakfast and she did most of it. Lunch and dinner at home included her crying in the kitchen till I told her to go to the chair till I got the meal ready. That is hard to do, but it is also hard to work when someone is standing by you crying. In the evening I asked if she knew where the container was that we take with us for picnic lunches. She got it immediately even though she had not seen it since before she got sick over a year ago. That told me she is very alert to what is going on even though she cannot communicate. A group of about 30 of us had a cruse on the lake with picnic lunch the next day.

We woke about 1:00 AM October 18th and had a nice conversation. She talked quite a bit. When we woke again about 7:00 she was sobbing. I dressed her.

The next day she told me what she wanted for breakfast. We ate dinner out and she ordered with less difficulty than usual. We discussed some things in the church bulletin which the choir director had written about old hymns. There was no big change the next three or four days. One day I did the laundry and did not put it in the dryer after it was washed. She reminded me to do that. Then she watched me as I made the bed. She said I put the bedspread on wrong.

About 9:00 PM it was obvious she was so tired she needed to go to bed. I asked if she wanted to go to bed and she said no. At 9:20 she was squirming in her chair, and it was obvious she wanted to get up. I told her I would help her if she would tell me she needed help. About ten minutes later she said "I guess I have to". Then I helped her to her feet and to bed.

When it was time to get dinner October 24th it was the old routine. I told her I welcomed her in the kitchen if she did not cry. She stayed near her chair and sobbed. When the meal was ready I literally fell apart. I cried more than she did.

I worked some in the yard the next afternoon. When I came in she was concerned about the rain which started just before I came in. I said she seems to feel better. She said "I dond't know."

We went to a board meeting after church and then to a special meeting at the church before the evening church service. It was a long day for her. She was very tired when she went to bed. I was reminded of a sign I saw on a ladies blouse that said "One day at a time is more than I can take." She was extremely silent the next day.

I had to dress her October 28th because she could not decide what to wear.

October 29th got better in the afternoon and we took a walk in the front yard. She talked some.

I told her I was in bad shape and plan to go for counseling when I can decide who to go to. I said I plan to go alone the first time and then want her to go with me. It was no surprise that she did not answer me.

November 1st I helped her start dressing and then walked out. She came out properly dressed in about thirty minutes. I asked what she wanted to eat and she did not tell me. When I gave her bacon and egg she said she told me she wanted cereal. She ate the bacon and egg with no protest. I worked in the yard about four hours so I suggested eating downtown. When I was ready to go she was near the door and said something about me wanting to go. That told me she wanted to go. She talked a little while we ate.

November 3rd, 2003. One year ago today a doctor told me he would give her four to six weeks to live. We thank our Lord she is with me today.

Alzheimer's, Depression and Dementia

I suggested going to a certain restaurant for dinner. She did not respond. Later she asked what we were doing for dinner. That made it clear she wanted to know if I wanted to eat out. We went out and she talked a little. When we got back she seemed better than she was in the early part of the day.

She woke in tears November 6th. I ate breakfast and went back and dressed her. She got to the kitchen about 8:45. After eating she did the back porch routine.

After dinner November 7th I said we should read the Sunday school lesson aloud as we had done before. She said something about not reading the scripture, but the other part of the Sunday school lesson as well. I suggested she read the commentary. Her reading was very good. What an improvewment. This has been one of the best days we have had in a long time. She stayed in the kitchen while I cleaned up after dinner, and she did not cry.

We had plans to go to a Couples Club dinner November 8th. She had no idea what she wanted to wear. I had to pick her clothes and put them on her. She was very quiet at the dinner although she spoke to some friends she had known before. She was very tired when we got home. I have told her I am writing notes about her illness, but I do not go into detail about it. Since she has always been such an alert lady it is surprising to me she never asks what I do when I go to the computer to write this. Prior to her illness she wanted to know everything that went on in our lives and there was very little I did not tell her. It is discouraging to see that the lady I spent so many wonderful years with is just not here anymore.

When I came in from the yard she was looking at my shoes. She thought I was wearing my dress shoes for yard work. I was not. Actually, I was wearing a pair I replaced recently. This and other observations by her cause me to think she notices and can do a lot of things she will not admit. It is probably that she just cannot communicate. Who can really tell?

Sunday morning as I was washing the dishes after breakfast she pealed a banana I had laid out for her. Then she said she did not know why she started that. After church we went out to eat and friends joined us. I had a nice visit with them, but she said practically nothing.

After dinner my sister called to tell us about my brother's wife who is seriously ill with cancer. Helen talked with her more than usual and seemed to be better after that.

I got up and ate breakfast alone. I intentionally let her stay in bed to see if she would get up by herself. She did not. I went back and put some of her clothes on her and walked out. I went back in about thirty minutes and finished dressing her. I asked what she wanted for breakfast and she finally told me. After eating she did the back porch routine without my saying anything about it.

She was in a pretty good mood when we woke the next morning, but in no hurry to dress. I told her she was on her own to dress and I would prepare her breakfast when she was ready. I looked in about fifty minutes later and she was almost dressed. We ate breakfast together. She was in fair shape when she went to bed. When I got her up the next day about 8:00 I told her she was on her own to dress. Since she dressed without my help yesterday I hoped she could do it today. I ate breakfast and went back about an hour later. She was up but had done practically nothing about dressing. I dressed her and she ate and then did the back porch routine. When the dryer sounded off to let me know it was ready to empty she called me.

She was really low all day. There was a ladies' meeting that night. Since she was so low I decided to say nothing about the meeting which was to start at 7:00 PM. After eating dinner I asked what she wanted for desert. She said there would be refreshments at the meeting. I took her to the meeting.

She was in not so bad a mood when she got up the next day but was in no hurry to dress. I did nothing to help her and she was almost dressed about fifty minutes later. She would not tell me what she wanted for breakfast.

She woke before I did November 14th. I had my back to her. She slapped me on the back at 7:00 AM and said it was time to get up. That was more like my wife than I had seen in a long time. When I got out of bed she was in tears. I had to put her clothes on her in spite of her protests. When she got to the kitchen she was better and she ate a normal breakfast. I had an appointment with the barber after lunch and she went with me. She talked some as we ate dinner at home. After dinner she was rather quiet till about 7:45 when she began to sob. About fifteen minutes later the sobbing was worse and I took her to the bath room. It must be horrible to need someone—even your spouse—to help you to the bathroom. Then together we read the Sunday school lesson for the next day. After dinner we went to the home of some friends to visit with missionaries who serve in West Africa.

Sunday, November 16th I asked her if she didn't think she was getting better. She said "well" and the after a pause she said "I hope so". Our evening service at the church was an informal meeting with missionaries from three different countries. She was very tired when we got home.

When we woke the next morning there was considerable pillow talk which made me feel great. When I went back to get her up things were completely different. She had no idea how to dress and after about ten minutes I dressed her in spite of her protests.

I decided to try another approach to get her to remember something from the past concerning her two previous breakdowns. I asked if she remembered the time of the year she had her first one. She said she did not. I asked if she remembered the name of the hospsital and she did not. She told me before she was age 24 when she had her first one. I asked if she was released from the hospital before or after her 25th birthday and she did not know. Her looks showed she was thinking very seriously while I was asking questions. Then I went to the kitchen to start lunch. She started crying.

She was in good spirits when we woke the next morning. When I helped her out of bed she was bad again. I helped her start dressing and walked out. One hour and five minutes later she was dressed when I went back to the bedroom. I told her to comb her hair and I would get breakfast. After eating I went to the TV to see a special program. I helped her get out of the chair and on her feet. A few minutes later I looked back and saw she was washing the dishes. After dinner I asked what board game she wanted to play. She did not answer. Shortly after 8:00 she indicated she wanted to get out of her chair. I asked what she was up to. She indicated she wanted to play a game. We played UpWords and she played a very good game. Even though she was tired when we finished I believe something like that helps her. Prior to her illness she read a lot. Now she reads practically nothing.

I had to dress her November 19th but it was not too difficult. She had plans to go to a ladies' meeting which started at 8:30. After I got her dressed she said two things

I put on her did not match and she was right. After we got in the car she said her panty hose looked bad. Things like that convince me she can think—at least about some things. On the way she said the meeting started at 9:00 but it started at 8:30 and when we got there many ladies were already there.

The next day she was sobbing at 5:00 AM and I took her to the bathroom. I got her up at 8:00. I told her I was about to eat and would prepare her breakfast when she dressed. I went back at 8:30 and dressed her. She went to the kitchen a few minutes later and ate a normal breakfast.

In the afternoon of November 21st I suggested we walk out front and with some hesitation she agreed. We walked to the front of the garage and she acted like she wanted to walk down the very steep drive. I had some doubts about this, but we walked down the drive and up the street. We walked about 65 or 70 normal steps and she said go back. We got back up the drive OK, but I was scared. I decided not to do this again till she got better. Dinner at home went OK. Actually, she was in the kitchen while I was cooking, and she did not cry. She seemed to be observing what I was doing with much interest. That was great. I made a mess of the meal. I critized it but she said very little.

She dressed herself the next morning but it took a long time for her to do it. When she came to the kitchen she was dressed properly except she had on shoes she would not ordinarily wear with that dress. I suggested she change shoes and she did it. She was very tired at bed time.

A few days ago I thought I was buying apple juice, but I got fruit punch instead. I do not remember her ever serving that, but I like it. I poured some for me, but not for her because I did not think she would like it. She said something about it, and said it tasted good the other day. I had not served it to her before. I poured some for her and she acted like she liked it. Oh that dementia. When she went to bed she was very tired. I mentioned a personal thing she said years ago and she said "I don't remember saying any dumb thing like that".

When she woke November 25th she was sobbing. I took her to the bathroom. Then she sobbed till she shook for a minute or two. She went back to bed till 7:45 when I got her up. I dressed her about 8:00. She had an appointment with her hair dresser and then we went to the Thanksgiving service.

The next day I told her it was up to her to get up and dress. I went to the kitchen and ate alone. After about forty-five minutes I went back and found her taking clothes out of the dirty clothes hamper. She said she was trying to find something to wear. I dressed her and then she ate.

When she woke November 27th she appeared to be in great shape. When she left the bathroom she started crying. I told her I would prepare her breakfast when she got dressed. After about an hour and a half I dressed her. She ate a normal breakfast and did the back porch routine. She said something about not having dinner at the church last night, and that Joe and Carolyn were bringing us a Thanksgiving dinner.

When she got up the next morning she said something about dressing "I can't—-", and I told her she could as I walked out. I dressed her in spite of her protests. I asked what she wanted for breakfast and she finally said "I guess I want cereal." She seemed better after breakfast as she usually does. I do not understand why she always seems to be better after breakfast when she always eats three good meals a day and we usually eat a snack just before bedtime.

This is just unbelievable for a lady who has always been as brilliant as she has. She is left handed and wears her watch on her right hand. When I got her out of bed this morning she had her watch on the fingers of her right hand. Dinner was the best meal we have had in some time because there were no tears. When I was preparing dinner she came to the kitchen, but did not cry. She asked about some things. We ate a good, pleasant meal and I told her I appreciated it.

I asked her several questions about the breakdown she had in 1960. She looked like she was trying to think, and I believe she was. She said she was in a fog. I asked about the times she visited friends in Chicago after moving to Indianapolis. She said she could not remember anything of importance. I said I appreciate her pastor suggesting she tell me about this and that she told me before we were married. I believe this was time well spent even though I did not get any answers. All through the discussuon she looked like she was trying to think, but could not come up with any answers.

Yesterday and the day before I suggested we go to Queen Willimena state park today and have dinner at the lodge. She would not say yes or no. I brought it up again today and we went. She was rather quiet, but did talk some. Prior to her illness we had enjoyed going there a few times.

After such a wonderful day yesterday it was about the same old routine November 29th. She was not able to dress herself.

The following morning she woke about 3:00 AM, turned on the light, and went to the bathroom without my help and without crying. It was a different story about 7:00 AM. While I prepared dinner she was in the kitchen, but did OK. She thought I was burning the chicken, but it turned out good. I popped some corn about 8:15 and she did her usual "oh no" but she ate some of it and seemed to enjoy it.

When I started to prepare dinner December 2nd she started crying in the kitchen. I told her she could stay in the kitchen only if she did not cry. She stood there a few minutes and then sat down. When I got dinner ready and we got to the table we had a rather pleasant meal.

She woke about 5:30 the next morning in low spirits. I helped her to the bath room and when she got back to bed I took her a glass of orange juice. At about 7:00 she said something about not being able to dress. I asked why and she did not reply. I helped her start dressing and then walked out. She got to the living room twenty or thirty minutes later fully dressed. She also brought out a water glass I always take to the bedroom for her at night. I do not remember her taking that to the kitchen before. She was more normal after breakfast. We went to the grocery and she made two or three good suggestions. Prior to her illness she did practically all the shopping. In the evening she properly told me I had not cleaned the top of the stove. Prior to her illness she read a lot, but now she reads practically nothing. I saw an article in the paper that I hoped would interest her. I showed it to her and she appeared to read it as well as other things in the paper. She made no comment.

Lunch went well. With a little help from me she got some turkey soup from the frig and put it in the microwave. I suggested this to help her build confidence. I suggested a game of UpWords and she said nothing. A few minutes later she indicated she wanted to get up, and I helped her up. Then she walked toward the table where we play games. Without saying anything she made it clear she wanted to play UpWords. She played a pretty good game till she got tired, and then she was very slow.

I went back about 7:20 AM December 5th and found her sitting on the side of the bed. I helped her get up and she did not know how to dress. She said "I can't" and I told her that was a vulgar word, and she should watch her language. I walked out. I worked in the yard some in the morning. When I came back she had gotten out of the chair and was on her feet.

Getting her dressed the next day was one of the worst times I have had yet. She could not dress herself and resisted everything I did. When she finally got to the breakfast table she was better. She ate a good meal last night and I can's believe she was that hungry. Just before lunch I learned I needed to go downtown. We ate lunch out and were gone about three hours. When I started dinner she went to the kitchen and started crying. I took her back to her chair. Before I finished she went back to the kitchen and did not cry so much. She asked some questions about the range and I believe I answered them.

When she woke December 7th she was crying and said she did not know what to put on. I walked out to see what she would do. In about thirty minutes she came to the kitchen properly dressed. This was less time than it usually takes.

Her cries woke me about 3:00 AM December 8th. I took her to the bathroom and her cry slowed down, and finally stopped. She said she had slept very little, if any. She got up about 7:30. I told her to dress herself and I walked out. She came to the kitchen properly dressed about an hour later. When I was getting lunch she commented on the looks of our frying pan. She thinks we need a new one. She got out of the chair without help and walked across the room.

That is great. I suggested going downtown for dinner and getting a new frying pan. She made no comment, but was ready to go. When we got to Sears she made the long walk across the store with no trouble. She seemed to know what she wanted, but when we got home she said she wished we had not bought that. She sat up later, and was in better shape when she went to bed. She said her nails needed trimming and I did that for her. While I was doing that we had a very nice conversation. We made no big plans, but we just had a nice talk. That went on till about midnight. Do you say that is no big deal? Just wait till you and your spouse cannot talk and see how wonderful it is to talk about anything.

When she woke the next morning it was about the same old routine. About 7:30 PM she indicated she wanted to get out of the chair, and I helped her up. She walked toward the table where we sit when we play games. It looked like she wanted to play UpWords, but at first she said no. After a pause she said she wanted to play and she played a fairly good game. She did not appear to be too tired till we finished, and then she was really tired.

The next morning it took a long time for her to say what she wanted to eat. She finally said she wanted cereal and she prepared it.

She spoke a few sentences of very good conversation when she woke December 11th and then it was over. After that it was another one of those days.

December 12th started off about as usual. We attended the Christmas program in the evening, and she was very tired when we got home. When she woke the next morning she seemed to be better, but when she got to the bathroom she started the old "I can't." I did the old routine and then went back and dressed her. After eating breakfast she indicated she wanted to get out of her chair. I wanted to see if she could get up without help. She got up on her own and walked to the other side of the sink. She put banana peelings in the garbage disposal and turned on the garbage disposal. We went downtown for dinner and saw a Christmas program at one of the best churches.

I got her up in the wee hours of the morning December 14th to go to the bath room. Then just before getting up time she turned on the light which is on her side of the bed, got up, and walked to the bathroom without my help. I had to dress her. This was Sunday and when we went out to eat after church she was able to order with less help. We had some conversation as we ate. When we got home we watched the news for a short time and she talked about that. I want to say wonderful, and then I ask myself what we can expect tomorrow.

She woke up sobbing the next morning because the ladies from the church we expected to stay with her while I was at a semimar could not do it, and we had to pay someone else. I tried to talk with her, but it did no good.

When I started to get dinner she started to cry. I said I would like for her to be with me in the kitchen, but only if she did not cry. She stood up and then sat down again. After we ate she got up and with no statement from either of us she walked to the other side of the sink, washed most of the dishes, and put them in the dish washer. She even dried the floor where she spilt some water while rinsing the dishes. I said I believe it is good for anyone to do something besides sit in a chair. I also said I did not say that just because I did not want to wash the dishes.

A new lady stayed with her Dec 17th and 18th while I went to a seminar. I was home both nights.

We had an appointment December 19th with the physician she has gone to for many years. He was pleased with her condition, and said her potassium was good. He does not know she has not taken the medicine he prescribed for about a month. I will talk with him about that at the proper time. I went to the grocery tonight and she put away some of the things I bought.

When I was ready to get dinner she said she did not know which pan to use to bake the chicken. She wanted to help me, but did not know what to do. It is hard to believe that my wonderful wife, who was such a good cook, is in that condition.

When we went out to eat after church she ordered the same thing I did with very little hesitation.

The next morning started off about as usual. I got out some of her underclothes and walked out. She came to the kitchen about thirty-five minutes later which was quicker than usual. She said she wanted cereal and then said I gave her too much. During the day she made two or three suggestions that told me she was thinking more clearly. She needed less help when she went to bed that night.

It took only about thirty minutes for her to dress the next day and that is quicker.

When we got up December 24th it was the old routine. I did a laundry and then ate. I went back to the bedroom and finished dressing her, and then prepared her breakfast. We went to the Christmas Eve service at the church and it was wonderful. She seemed better when she got up about 7:50 Christmas day and she did not say the old "I can't". I walked out and went back about thirty minutes later and dressed her. We ate together. We were invited out for Christmas dinner with four couples. It was great, but she was so quiet.

There was nothing too different about December 26th and 27th. December 28th was out 41st wedding anniversary. She seemed OK till she got out of bed and then could not decide what to put on. She objected to what I triesd to put on her. I was both angry and in tears. When we drove downtown for the anniversary dinner I cried a lot while driving. We were both calmed down some when we got to the restaurant. I asked several questions about what happened before her previous breakdowns. I believe she was really trying to think, but was not able to remember anything. Since she could remember nothing about the years between 1943 and 1947 I said I believed something bad happended to her then. We were both in bed about 11:15 PM. We had more communication starting about 11:30 than we have had recently. We went to sleep about midnight.

About 9:00 PM December 29th I jokingly suggested she get on the trampoline. She got on and did 185 bounces with me holding her arm. She stayed up till 10:00. We talked a lot and a big part of it was the "lost" years between 1943 and 1947.

She walked to the kitchen December 30th after I ate. She had the frying pan in her hand and I showed her how to turn on the stove. She broke the egg and put it in the pan. I put the bacon in the frying pan. She poured her juice. That probably sounds so simple to you who have not been through it. I call it a great improvement.

She talked when we woke December 31st. Then when she got up she did not know how to dress. She prepared her cereal and poured her juice. I prepared her toast. We ate dinner at the church New Year's Eve service.

When we got up January 1st, 2004 she started the old "I can't" about dressing. I told her she could and she would dress herself. She came to the kitchen fully dressed sooner than I expected. We ate breakfast together and she did the back porch routine. We watched the Parade of Roses. After lunch she got up on her own and washed the dishes. She was in the kitchen while I got dinner and cried very little. She questioned what I did to heat the oven and I explained it to her. After eating I told her this is one of the best meaks we have had recently.

She has always been weight conscious. When I got up January 3rd I got on the bathroom scales and saw I was down a couple of pounds. I turned the scales where she could see them and got on them again. I said I was down and she said "what about it?"

She came to the kitchen at 8:25 January 6th. I did not leave my chair, but asked what she wanted for breakfast and if she wanted me to prepare it. She prepared cereal and I prepared her toast. In the evening I asked if there was anything that happened at the hospital or nursing home that stood out in her mind. She looked like she was trying to think, but never said anything. I asked about certain things, but she was silent.

She came out about twenty-five minutes after I walked out January 7th and we had breakfast together. There was nothing too different about the remainder of the day.

I told her I was concerned about the four years she could not remember. Considerable conversation on this subject produced nothing new.

She seemed to be better when we woke Sunday, January 11th, till she got out of bed. She was not able to dress. I had to pick her clothes and force dress her. After church she was very sad when we went out to eat. She ate a good meal, but said she was not able to eat all they put on her plate. I suggested going for a drive in the scenic mountains. She said we should not. I asked why not, and she did not seem too opposed, so we did it. We had some conversation.

In the afternoon of January 12th I cleaned out the refrigerator and threw out some things that had been there too long. She was sitting across the room, but she asked why I threw out something I had just purchased. I had not done that. I suggested going downtown about 4:45. Thirty-five minutes later she replied. We ate downtown.

She woke about 4:00 AM January 13th and when I took her to the bathroom the crying ceased. We woke again about 7:00 and I got up and ate. I got her up about 8:00, and told her dressing was up to her. About forty-five minutes later she had her underclothes on and was looking at a certain pair of slacks. I helped her get them off the hanger, and walked out again. She finished dressing. When she got to the kitchen she said she wanted cereal, and she prepared it. She cried in the kitchen while I got lunch. She was in the kitchen while I prepared dinner, but did not cry much. I messed up the meal I was cooking. That was my fault.

She went to a ladies' breakfast January 14th that started at 8:45. I wanted her to go. She told me practically nothing about the meeting. Lunch at home went OK. After lunch I showed her how I was preparing some ribs for dinner that night. Together we opened the oven and looked at them about 3:00.

January 17th was not too different till about 4:30 when I started talking about going downtown to see and hear Dino. I had mentioned this before, but she had not said yes or no. She liked him when we saw him before her illness. I believe she enjoyed it. We got home about 10:15 and she was not too tired.

She helped me get lunch January 19th. She actually did some of the work and I believe that helps give her some confidence in her ability.

We have been going to a series of four evening meetings, two of which are still to go. Last night she was so tired when she got home and I wonder if this is too much for her. I also wonder if staying home by ourselves and "looking at the four walls" is too much. While eating dinner I asked if she wanted to go tonight. Several minutes later I asked again, and she said she was trying to decide. She never said, in words, what she wanted to do. While I was washsing the dishes she went to the cloaset and got her coat. We went. On the way to the meeting I said her indecision, such as taking so long to decide whether to go, reminds me of what I have seen through the years. I said she usually makes good decisions, but takes a long time to do it. She disagreed with me.

We woke about 7:25 January 23rd and she got out of bed and to the bathroom without my help. I did not offer to help her because I wanted to see if she could and would do it. About an hour later I had to dress her.

Lunch did not go well the next day as she cried in the kitchen. I told her how wonderful it would be if she would talk with me. She said "I dond't know what to say". I said we could talk about the things we have done in the past or, better, what we hope for in the furure. She said nothing more.

About 5:00 PM I asked her to join me in the kitchen and pick what she wanted me to cook. She came to the kitchen but made no suggestions. She only cried. I lost it again. I said again it is hard to be deserted—in the same house, but a million miles apart. That was not nice of me. Dinner was not a pleasure.

When we woke January 25th she talked a little, but she could not dress. I had a board meeting and she went with me. On the way home she made two or three comments I call normal small talk. That was encouraging. When we got home she mentioned some things that came up at the meeting. I felt like I was coming down with a cold and drank a lot of grapefruit juice, which I have done before for the same reason. She asked why I was drinking so much juice. That was great because I have heard her ask the same question before her illness. About 9:30 PM she said in a very clear voice she should go to bed.

The next day started off bad, but she rode the bike about half a mile. Her normal ride is about a quarter mile. That is further than I remember her ever riding it, and I told her that was good.

One night we had a heart to heart talk after going to bed. I told her how much it hurts me for her to cry so much. Actually, I did most of the talking. She said very little and seemed to have at least some agreement with what I said. She was ready to go to bed about 9:50. When I got up a little before 8:00 the next morning she said "I don't know what to do". I walked out after getting her started. When I went back at least half an hour later she had done nothing about dressing. I dressed her in spite of her protests. We had to go downtown and were gone about two hours. That and the other Wednesday activities was just too much for her. It was just not a good day.

When it was time to get dinner I asked her to come to the kitchen to see what I was doing. She was such a great cook before she got sick. I showed her such simple things as how to open a can of chicken and dumplings with an electric can opener, put them in the dish and in the microwave, and how to set the microwave. She started crying, but I let her stay in the kitchen. It was my desire that she learn to do some things which I am sure she wants to do. We had a fairly good meal. It just does not seem possible that I understand more about the kitchen than she does.

When we woke January 30th she talked quite a bit and seemed to be in better spirits. When she got up she showed signs of the old depression. I walked out, and when I went back I found her dressed quicker than I expected. We had breakfast together. She said it was cold outside, but she did the bike ride and then walked some in the house. That night we got a call telling us my younger brother who has cancer was not expected to live more than a few days. That brought more tears.

She walked toward the kitchen January 31st and said she did not know what to do about getting lunch. About 2:20 she commented about the red lights on the stove. I asked her to go to the kitchen with me, and I showed her how the lights work. We had a fairly good dinner and she talked some.

Monday morning she woke me by rubbing my back. She has done this several times lately. She did not seem to be able to dress, so I started dressing her. I was interrupted by a phone call and when the call was over she was almost dressed.

She woke me about 5:00 AM February 4th and said the stove was making noises. I did not believe her, but I checked and found that after cooking dinner I had not turned off the oven. I told her she was right. I looked in about 8:50 and saw she was well on the way dressing. She got to the kitchen about 9:00. I just sat in the chair and did not even ask what she wanted to eat. She prepared cereal and then poured orange juice. As she started to sit down I asked if she wanted toast. She put bread in the toaster and asked me to butter it for her which I did. She finished eating and then put the dishes in the dish washer. She watched as I heated the casserole for lunch. She was confused about how long it would take to heat. Lunch was very nice. After eating dinner she went to another room and was out fifteen or twenty minutes. When she came back to the living room she said she wanted to apologize. I asked what for, and she said for exploding earlier. I took that to mean what happened when I came back from the grocery before dinner. Then we had a good conversation. Some of this was serious, but some was just small talk. This has been one of our best evenings recently.

She continues to sit up a little later than she did which indicates she is feeling better.

I opened a can of tuna salad for lunch. I went to the chair and asked her to put the tuna on the toast. She seemed to enjoy doint that. Just think. She was such a great cook for so long. Lunch went well. About 5:15 I asked her to put some frozen chicken in the oven. It was a major job for her to decide which of the four pieces in the box to put in the pan to cook. She finally did it and put the pan in the oven. Twenty minutes later she was still standing by the stove. Dinner went well.

February 10th started out like a bad day. I did the usual and then walked out. I looked back a time or two and saw nothing to encourage me. Then much to my pleasant surprise I saw her standing by the stove trying to figure out how to fry bacon and egg. I showed her how to do it and she ate. At lunch time I asked what she wanted . In a crying voice she said we were out of bread. We ate lunch out and then I went to the grocery alone. When I got back I showed her what I purchased, and she was pleasant. I asked her to come to the kitchen while I prepared dinner and I showed her everything I was doing. We had a pleasant time. I am not speaking of the food when I say we had the best meal we have had recently. The atmosphere was very good and we had much more two way conversation. I helped her out of the chair at 10:45, and she prepared for bed without my help.

Next morning she was in the kitchen at 8:40 with very little help from me.

She prepared her ceral and orange juice. I asked if she wanted toast and she indicated she did not. Then she said she guessed she needed something else. I prepared her toast. Then she did the back porch routine.

The next day started bad. I walked out and when I came back forty-five minutes later she had done nothing about dressing. I walked out again, and she finished dressing. She told me what she wanted to eat. We went to the bank and grocery after lunch. As we were going home she said she had not gotten anything for the baby shower she was going to that night. When we got home she sat down at the table to wrap it. An hour or so later she said she did not know what to do. This is the type of thing she always enjoyed before. I helped her wrap it. I took her to the shower and picked her up about 9:45.

I opened a can of chicken salad for lunch February 13th and suggested she put it on toast. She did it. I put the laundry in the washer in the morning. Just before lunch she asked if I had put it in the dryer. I had not. When they were dry she carried some of them to the closet and volunteered to help me make the bed.

I asked her to go to the kitchen when I got ready to get dinner February 14th. She listened to what I told her, but she was unable to do anything on her own. We had a pleasant time, but it is so sad to see her in that condition. I noticed she was reading the scripture about 8:00 PM. After she stopped reading we had a good discussion about what she had read and other scripture. She stayed up till 10:00 to see a musical program both of us enjoy.

Due to severe weather conditions there were no church services Sunday, February 15th. When she got to the kitchen she did not tell me what she wanted to eat, but prepared her own cereal. I asked if she wanted toast and she said she guessed so. She never seems to be sure—so often she says she "guesses" she needs something. Weather conditions were better by noon so we went out to eat. I asked where she wanted to go and she did not reply. I drove to a place she always enjoyed before her illness. She said she did not know why we had to go there.

She could not dress herself February 16th and strongly resisted my efforts to dress her. Due to snow on the porch she did not do the bike ride. As I was preparing lunch she started crying in the kitchen. I put her back in her chair. When I got certain things together I asked her to come back and fix the sandwiches. She did that and seemed to enjoy it. While preparing dinner I showed her how to put some frozen chicken in the oven to bake.

She got out of bed by herself the next morning. I did not offer to help her because I wanted to see what she could do. We ate together.

As I walked out February 19th I said her clothes were in the closet and it was up to her to dress. When she got to the kitchen I said nothing about preparing her breakfast and she said nothing. She prepared her cereal and talked a little. I gave her two choices for dinner at home or go out. She said nothing. I decided on chow mein. She said she did not know how to prepare that. She stayed in the kitchen and watched as I prepared it. She said I was putting too much on the plates. When she ate hers I put more on each plate. She protested, but she ate her part. Then we ate ice cream and graham crackers. The next two days were about the old routine.

Sunday, February 22nd, I had to literally force her to let me start dressing her. Then I walked out and she finished dressing in a fairly short time. I asked what she wanted for breakfast, and she finally said she guessed she had better have an egg. I asked why she "had better have" and she did not reply. She ordered dinner at the restaurant with less difficulty than she usually has.

We started talking about how long we had lived in our present house and the three prior houses. We have been in the present house just over eighteen years. Neither of us could remember how long we were in the prior houses. I went to my file and got a picture of our prior house when it was for sale and our present house when we purchased it. She looked at them closely—especially the one where we now live. There was conversation and that was great. Her mind was working very good. She stayed up till 10:30 and did not appear to be too tired.

When she got up the next morning she started to shower and then was worried about what it would do to her hair, which she had done yesterday. I asked what her shower cap was for. She showered.

Lunch February 25th started off with her crying in the kitchen, and I put her back in her chair. When I was ready to "put the sandwiches together" I asked her to do it. She said she did not know what to do with the ham. I told her I would do it. I just cannot believe this has happened to my wonderful wife. She washed the dinner dishes without a word from me. This is good.

She was ready to eat about 9:00 the next morning. When we sat down to eat she told me this is the day they pick up the garbage. I told her it was ready, but I had not put it out on the street yet. Breakfast went very well.

We had an invitation to have dinner with six couples who were all friends of ours. She talked very little. The group sat around a table and told about what they did before moving here. When I told my part about how we met she talked more than any other time in the evening. She was very tired when we got home.

She went to the bathroom about 10:15 PM and I thought she was going to bed. I stayed up to do some things I wanted to do after she went to bed. She called me about 11:00. I found she was in the bathroom, and not ready for bed.

I got her up about 8:00 the next morning and told her she needed some breakfast. I finally got her dressed and she got to the kitchen about 9:00. She could not tell me what she wanted to eat. She went to the stove and acted like she wanted an egg and bacon, but did not know how to prepare it. I did it for her. She cried when I did it. That was probably because it hurt her so bad to know she could no longer do the most simple things.

She woke March 2nd and turened on the light to go to the bathroom. She patted me on the back and said it was three o'clock. We got up about the usual time, and she got to the kitchen about 9:00. She went to the stove like she wanted an egg and bacon. Then she got a cereal bowl. After eating I helped her up from her chair. Then she went to the sink and washed the dishes. Then she picked up a banana and was having trouble peeling it. She said something to the effect she should not eat that. I pealed it and she ate it. I suggested the back porch routine and she did it. I asked if she wanted to go to the kitchen and see what we had for lunch. She was in the chair and started whimpering. I told her to sit there and I would get lunch. I opened a can of tuna and put bread in the toaster. Then I asked her to come to the kitchen and put the tuna on toast. She did it. I continue to ask her to do simple things like that. I believe it was helpful to her.

A client came in. It had been raining and he insisted on taking off his shoes so he would not leave tracts. After he left she insisted he had been here before. She said she remembered his taking off his shoes like he did today. He was a new client and I had never seen him before. Oh that dementia.

When she got up the next day she said she did not have anything to wear. I asked what all that stuff was in her closet. She seemed to have a cold. When she heard me calling her doctor's office she said "oh no". I told her I had to do it.

She was squirming in her chair and I could tell she needed to go to the bathroom. I told her if she would speak to me and tell me she needed help I would help her. She did not speak, but finally got up without my help. After we went to bed I tried to tell her how much it hurts me for her never to talk with me. She just laid there and stared at me. Oh how lonely it gets.

This is her 87th birthday. I mentioned this at least twice a few days ago and she had very little to say. Today I asked where she wanted to go for her birthday dinner. I mentioned the Red Lobster, one of her favorite places. Quite a long time later she said she wanted to go there. I ordered and she asked for the same. I thought that was because she was not able to choose. She changed to vegetables instead of the baked potato I ordered. When the meal came out she said she never dreamed there would be so much food. She was not able to eat all of her meal. When we got home I went to sleep in the chair. She woke me at 10:30. It was later than she should have stayed up.

When we woke about 5:30 March 10th she talked with me like my wife of many years ago. What a wonderful time for a few minutes. We went back to sleep and woke about an hour later. It was not the same. She was not crying, but had all the other symptoms of her current problems.

I took her to a ladies' meeting that started at 7:00 PM and picked her up at 9:00. On the way home I asked about the main theme of the meeting and she told me. That was an improvement. She seemed to be much better till we went to bed.

She was whimpering when she woke March 14th and then cried. She said something about not having anything to wear, or not knowing what to wear.

She has been eating later, but we needed to leave for church a little after 9:00. She resisted when I dressed her, but was better when we got to the kitchen. What can I say? It seems like a replay of the old routine. I am thankful she is alive and able to walk on her own, but it would be so great to see her in her right mind for more than such a short period at a time. She has always been such a brilliant lady.

I did not ask what she wanted for breakfast, but tried something new. When I put it in front of her and asked if it was fit to eat she said she quessed I was trying to make an omelet. I was not nice about her response.

We were awake about 4:00 AM March 16th. I have noticed several times lately when we are awake in the wee hours of the morning she is more alert. She was always what I call a night owl. She did not like to get up early. I told her about what I called a crazy dream of seeing the house where we lived before. She said I had told her about that before.

About 4:00 PM I asked her to go to the kitchen to see what we had for dinner. She went, but seemed to have no idea what to cook. I put some things in the oven that would take about two hours to bake. I left the kitchen for about an hour. When I went back she was still there, and I think she had been there since I left. She stayed till dinner was ready to eat. I went to sleep on the couch about 8:00 PM. When I woke at 10:20 I did not see her. She was in the bathroom getting ready for bed. She said she called me but I did not respond.

I got up about 7:00 March 20th and told her getting up and dressing was up to her. I wanted to see what she would do. Later she told me she needed help. I said I would help her later. Shortly after that I helped her start dressing and walked out again. She got to the kitchen about 9:00. With my help, like telling her to pour the juice and put bread in the toaster, she helped get breakfast. She stayed in the kitchen as I cooked dinner. I showed her as much as possible. It continues to seem impossible that I could show my wonderful wife who was such an excellent cook anything about the kitchen.

She was awake when I went back to the bedroom about 7:30. She said she could not find anything to put on. I said she could and she yelled out very loud "I can't". She had never yelled before. I said "you can" and I walked out. I went back at 7:55 and found her in the bathroom. I set a glass of orange juice before her and left again. Shortly after 9:00 she was in the kitchen with no more help from me.

We ate dinner downtown but the main idea was to see The Passion of the Christ. I was advised the film might be too much for her. She took it OK but told me it was hard for her to watch it. She talked quite a bit before and after the movie.

Since I could not sleep I went to the living room to read about 4:30 AM. She came in about 5:00 to check on me.

When I was ready to prepare dinner I asked her to go to the kitchen and tell me what she wanted. It was the same sad story. She could not decide, started crying, and I took her back to the chair till dinner was ready. That is so discouraging. I suggested a game of UpWords about 7:30. Twenty minutes later she indicated she wanted to get up and I helped her up. The way she walked and where she walked told me she wanted to play.

The next day I went back at 7:50 and found her sitting on the side of the bed. She said she could not go out there like this. I helped her to the bathroom and walked out. Since she has dressed herself the last two days I believe it is good to see if she will do it more often. She was in the kitchen at 9:15. This is the third day she has dressed herself and today was about thirty minutes earlier. She prepared her own cereal and I prepared the toast. I told her it looks like she eats cereal every day, but I like more variety. Compared to what it has been recently lunch was wonderful. We went to the church dinner. While sitting at the table she chuckled at something that was said. I had not heard a laugh like that in a long time. When we got home things were quiet, but pleasant.

She dressed March 26th with no help from me and got to the kitchen about 10:00. After lunch she pointed to the dishes and said she did not know what to do with them. I told her she could wash them or I would. She started washing them and I finished the job.

Next day she said something about not having anything to wear, or not knowing how to dress. I told her to do what she did yesterday, and I walked out. I did a few things and then got a phone call. When I looked in at 9:30 she was sitting at the breakfast table and had almost finished eating. I said I had to go to the grocery and I would like for her to go with me. Later she came out and asked if I was ready to go. It was a pleasant trip.

At the dinner table I asked if she would mind if I wrote her nephew and asked about what he knew that might be a burden on her mind. She said she would prefer I did not. I did not tell her I wrote him about a month ago and got a reply yesterday. I asked her about her trouble with her half brother and his trouble with his step-mother—her mother. Her answer agreed with what her nephew had written me, but she did not seem to suspect I got the idea from her nephew. He told me some things she did not tell me. In fact, she did not tell me anything. She just answered a question or two I asked. I knew I should go slow on this.

The next day, Sunday, I had to force her to let me start dressisng her to get started on time. I made certain she did not see the letter from Don, her nephew, until I had carefully read and considered it. He told about actions of his father, her older half brother, including his close association with his father who was also Helen's father, his disagreements with his step mother (Helen's mother), and a certain remark her half brother made at their father's funeral. He had said something to the effect that since his father was dead there was no reason for him to come back to visit. I showed her Don's letter this afternoon and she read it carefully, after reading the letter I had written Don. We spent about an hour with her reading the letters and our discussion. She could not remember what he said after the funeral. She could not even remember going to the funeral, but she did remember going to the viewing.

After we went to bed the next night she brought up the subject of Don's letter which she read yesterday. She did not remember whose funeral it was he referred to. I told her it was her father's funeral. We had an interesting discussion about this and his life as reported by his son Don in his letter. I went to my files and got his letter and she read it again.

She got up about 3:00 PM April 1st and went to the other room to tell me UPS had delivered a package. It seems to me she can get up when she wants to. There was more than the normal communication tonight. She was up till 11:00 PM and seemed quite content till she went to bed.

We got a call April 2nd from out of town friends who were visiting in the village. They invited us to have dinner with them at a restaurant. She talked with them a little, but it was not what could be called a normal visit for her part.

I got up at 6:45 Sunday, but did not suggest she get up till later. When she got up I walked out. I went back later, helped her start dressing, and walked out again. A few minutes later she came to the kitchen and asked what I ate for breakfast. I said I had not eaten. She asked what I wanted. I told her either an egg or cereal. Then I said it would be easier for her to fix cereal. I suggested she do it and she did. I prepared the toast and she poured the juice. That was the best meal we have had in a long time. After eating I went to the computer and found the time had changed. We missed Sunday school.

I suggested reading the Sunday school lesson for next Sunday. I read the scripture part and she read the commentary from the Sunday school book. This lasted about half an hour and was very pleasant. She was very alert.

After the good study last night I wanted another one tonight. After studtying a book on the movie Passion of the Christ I handed it to her and asked her to look at it. She studied it quite a while till the 700 Club came on. Then we watched the 700 Club till it ended at 11:00.

The next day started about the same old routine, but got better. She got to the kitchen about 9:45, and was wearing one of her pretiest blouses which she had not worn in a long time.

She came out about 9:15 April 8th after dressing with no help from me. At 10:00 she reminded me I had a chiropractic appointment. I did have one, but it was later than she thought.

The next day she chose not to go to the grocery with me. When I got back I asked her to come to the kitchen to see what I purchased. She started crying when she got to the kitchen and I told her to get out of the kitchen. I took her to the bedroom and told her she could come back to the living room when she quit crying. In less than five minutes I went back and asked her to come back. She came back and did not cry. This probably sounds brutal if you have not been "over the road".

Lunch April 12th went about as usual. I am now convinced that when she helps—like putting meat on the toast and pouring drinks—it helps her a lot. I really believe she cries because she is so heartbroken because she cannot do the things she always did so well and enjoyed so much. My reactions to her crying are not always proper, but it really hurts me to try to work with her standing nearby crying. What can I do? While I was preparing dinner she cried in the kitchen. I made her go to the chair. In less than five minutes I asked her to come back and set the table and pour the drinks. She did it. We had a pleasant dinner.

April 13th I told her I would like her opinion on something and she did not reply. After repeating this a time or two I showed her a letter I had written her doctor stating she had not taken her medicine in several months. I told her I wanted to show that to her doctor when we see him in about two weeks. She seemed to study the letter, but did not say a word. I did see some tears in her eyes, but that was no surprise.

Prior to her illness she had a slight problem with hair growing on her chin but she, being a perfectionest, always took care of it. Many times afttr she got sick I had to ask her to take care of that. Today she took care of that without me saying a word. I consider that an improvement.

When we woke this morning I mentioned that she said a pair of pants I wore yesterday were worn out. I asked if she thought I should throw them out. She said yes, but she did not know what I would wear. She has been worried about her not having anything to wear, and now she is worried about the same for me. Actually, both of us have plenty clothes. We attended a couples club dinner. It was the old routine. She seemed to enjoy it, but said practically nothing to the people who sat at the table with us.

She came to the kitchen while I was preparing dinner and started whimpering. I insisted she set the table so she would have something to do and the whimpering almost stopped. Dinner went fairly well. As I washed the dishes she stood on the other side of the sink and watched me.

I got her up at 7:15 because she had an appointment to give blood for a doctor's appointment. She said "I can't" but I told her she could. She yelled "I can't" as I walked out. She was properly dressed shortly after 8:00. That was quicker than she has dressed in a long time.

Lunch and dinner went quite well. Consideriang what life has been for many months there was considerable conversation today. She chose to sit up till 11:00 and seemed to enjoy it, and talked with me a little.

It is getting to be a more or less routine prosedure that when I am preparing lunch or dinner and she cries in the kitchen I force her to leave the kitchen. Then in three to five minutes I ask her to come back and set the table, or do some other simple jobs. She does it without crying. I hate to do this, but it works.

We watched gospel music on TV till 10:00, and then I helped her out of the chair. She walked to the bathroom without my help.

After she finally got dressed Sunday, April 25th, things went OK. I had a board meeting downtown in the afternoon and she went with me.

The next morning she dressed herself and came out about 9:30. She was rather slow deciding on what she wanted to eat, but finally decided on egg and bacon which I prepared for her.

She came out properly dressed about 8:30 April 27th and asked what I ate. I told her I ate cereal because I was too lazy to fry an egg. I said I would fry her an egg if she wanted it. She looked around and then prepared her cereal.

After eating she did the back porch routine. We saw her doctor at 11:30 and he was pleased with her condition. He said her cholesterol was bad, but he said he did not recommend the medicine that was available for that. He said she has authorities, but indicated that goes with old age. After he gave us his report I showed him my detailed statement showing she had not taken any medicine in more than five months. After the doctor read my statement he walked out and the last thing he said was "no more medications". My personal opinion is that he knew he had been caught overdosing her for years. She always thought he was a good doctor. I always had reservations, but had no facts I could tie down.

When we left the doctor's office I asked where she wanted to eat lunch and she told me. I cannot remember when she told me where she wanted to eat out before. She was in the kitchen when I prepared dinner, and she made some good suggestions. That was great. Thank the Lord. She was some better the following day and dressed herself.

The following day I told her I had done the washing and the clothes were in the dryer. She said all her clothes were in the washing, and she had nothing to put on. I said she had other clothes in the closet. She got to the kitchen about 9:30. After eating she said she did not know how to get the egg and stuff off her plate. I told her it could be done with soap and water. She said something about when the frying pan would be washed. I told her I wash that every time I wash the dishes. I believe she is getting better, but things like that concern me. She was in the kitchen most of the time when I prepared dinner, and dinner went quite well.

When we woke April 30th she was in a good mood, and then she started crying. I went back about 7:30 and took her orange juice. She made the usual statement about not knowing what to put on. When I went back about 8:40 she was dressed, and had almost finished making the bed. This was the first time she had made the bed by herself since she came home from the nursing home more than ten months ago. After eating she made some helpful suggestions about what I was doing in the kitchen. It turned out to be a better day.

When I went back May 1st she was getting clothes from the dirty clothes hamper. When I asked why she said she did not have any others. I forced her to go to the closet and get clean clothes. Later I went back and helped her dress. She got to the kitchen about 10:00.

Sunday afternoon, May 2nd, I called some friends about a three day meeting like we had attended before she got sick. After I hung up she said she did not want to go.

The next day I went back about 8:30 and found her in the bathroom. I handed her a bra and she hit me with the bra. No injury, of course. She got to the kitchen about 10:00 and after eating she did the back porch routine.

It was the old routine to start May 6th She got to the kitchen at 9:50. She took several minutes to decide what she wanted to eat, but finally said egg and bacon. She put the bacon and egg in the frying pan. We had a very pleasant dinner and I told her that after eating.

May 7th she was standing by her closet and said "I can't". I said "you can". She said "I won't". I said "you will" and walked out. The yelling is fairly new. I asked what she wanted to eat and she finally said she guessed she wanted an egg. She got out the egg and bacon and put them in the frying pan.

She got to the kitchen about 10:00 May 8th with considerable help from me. There was nothing too unsual about the day.

I had to force dress her Sunday, but after she finally got dressed things went about normal.

Monday after dinner I told her I had to go to the grocery. She chose not to go with me. When I got back she went to the kitchen and started crying. I told her to go back to her chair. Before she got to the chair I told her she could come back if she would not cry. She came back and did not cry so much.

She seemed to be in good shape when she woke May 11th. I went back about 8:15 and saw her standing by the closet with stockings in hand as if she did not know what to do with them. Much to my surprise she had made the bed and it looked great. I helped her put on her underclothes. She finished dressing and fried her bacon and egg with little help from me.

After she got to the kitchen May 12th I went back and saw she had made the bed—the second day in a row. This is pot luck night at the church dinner. I prepared some ribs which I like, but the last time I served them at home she complained. At my request she tasted them at home, but made no comment. I told her she could eat other people's cooking. She took some of them at church, as well as other people's cooking. She made no comment. The bowl was empty after dinner so somebody ate them. There was more than the usual pillow talk after we went to bed.

The next day she got to the kitchen about 9:30 and she made the bed before that. Last night we got Rick Warren's book The Purpose Driven Life from the church library. There are forty chapters in it and the author recommends reading one chapter a day and thinking about it before reading the next. She read the first chapter out loud last night. Today at about 4:30 she read chapter two out loud. I went to the grocery alone after dinner. When I got back she helped put away the groceries and it was a pleasant experience. This has been a better day.

After considerable stalling May 15th she decided she wanted bacon and egg and she prepared it. Then she washed her dishes. As she was walking toward her chair

I told her I need her help and she is the only one who can help me. She just stared at me. I told her, again, I do not know how much longer I can live when she does not cooperate with me. I asked if she is willing to help. She grunted something I could not understand. She seemed to be saying she was willing to help, but I could not understand her. That probably sounds brutal to anyone except me. I do not want to hurt her. I want to help her. Who knows what I should do?

I got her off her chair at 10:25 and said she had not done her bike ride the last two days. She did the bike ride. I told her I was going to a political meeting at 11:00 and wanted her to go with me. At 10:55 she said she would go with me. The meeting was interesting to me. She said nothing for or against it. We have a record of being in agreement with almost all such things.

Sunday morning we went to a special meeting at the mission. I never know how long it will take her to dress so I got her up early. She was properly dressed at 7:55, much quicker than I expected. She made the bed four days in a row, but today and yesterday she did not do it. Breakfast together was nice.

The next morning she finished dressing and ate much earlier than usual. At 11:15 I told her I was going after gas for the lawn mower and asked her to go with me. I put some gas in the can to rinse it out and the attendant took it to pour it out. When he brought back the can she said it was not the same can I gave him. She said it was a different color. It was the same can. Is this the dementia?

I went to the bathroom about 2:00 PM May 21st expecting to find her there. She was making the bed. Sunday, May 23rd, she stumbled walking on a level floor at the church. I was holding her arm, so she did not fall. She woke me at 3:15 AM May 24th to tell me she was dizzy.

We woke about 6:00 AM May 25th and we talked quite a bit. She went back to sleep and got to the kitchen about 9:20. After she ate I went back to the bedroom and found she was making the bed. She was having trouble getting the sheets straight so I helped her. We played UpWords and finished just before 10:00 PM. I questioned whether she should stay up to see the 700 Club, but she chose to see it. She did not appear to be so tired when we went to bed.

Starting May 27th was about the old routine with her getting to the kitchen about 9:50. About 4:30 PM I suggested she walk to the mail box with me and then we walked up the street and back to the house. This was a round trip of about two hundred yards, and included walking down, and back up, a very steep drive. I held her arm very carefully all the way and she had no trouble. The day went quite well. I asked if she thought she would be OK if I went to a men's prayer and Bible study breakfast tomorrow morning before she normally gets up. She said very little, but did not object. I left the next morning about 7:00 and got back at 9:10. I got her out of bed soon after getting back. About 1:30 I asked if she would like to take a trip and I mentioned Mount Nebo. She asked me if I was ready to go about fifteen minutes later. While eating dinner she came out with three smiles like I had not seen in far too long a time. She was more like my wife of several years ago. After we got home she admitted she thinks she is getting better.

When she got up May 31st she said she did not know what to put on. I told her it was too cold not to put on anything, especially if she went outside. She slapped me twice for saying that and I laughed as I walked out. She was ready for breakfast about 11:00. I ate much earlier and we ate lunch about 1:00.

I went back about 8:35 June 1st and got her up. Half an hour later she was not dressed. She got to the kitchen about 10:30. Lunch and dinner went quite well. In the afternoon I asked her to go to the grocery with me, but since she did not answer I went alone.

When we woke about 6:00 June 2nd she was sobbing. The sobbing ceased and she went back to sleep. She was awake about 8:40 and I got her up. The first thing she said was she did not know what she was going to do. I told her the first thing to do was to put on a smile. She went to the bathroom, but did not put on the smile. Lunch was not good. She thought I was fixing too much for lunch. After the sandwich I asked if she wanted cantaloupe or something else. She did not answer. I cut my cantaloupe and she said she did not want that. I helped her up and she got ice cream. When I started washing dishes she came to the sink, and started crying. I told her if she had to cry she could do it in the other room.

About 6:45 June 4th she reminded me I wanted to go to the men's prayer and Bible study. When I got back at 8:55 I insisted she get up. I had to start dressing her and then I walked out. She was in the kitchen about 10:20. While I was preparing dinner she cried so much in the chair I took her to the bedroom where I could not hear her. I told her she could come back when she quit crying. At the dinner table I cried more than she did. I told her the choices for desert and she did not answer. I got up and got mine. After considerable time she got up and got ice cream for herself. I told her June 4th I plan to use her system and speak to her so seldom it appears I am ignoring her.

When the laundry was ready to take out of the dryer June 6th she got up without help and helped me take clothes out of the dryer. She carried some of them to the closet where we keep them. That goes along with the way things have been lately. When she finally gets out of bed, dresses, and eats, she seems much better. She seemed better when we went to bed.

I went back about 8:40 the next day and insisted she get up and eat. I went back later and helped her start dressing. She got to the kitchen just before 10:00. When I was getting lunch she cried so much I took her to the bedroom. No more than five minutes later I went back and got her. She put the sandwiches together and did not cry. We had some very interesting conversation after eating. We did the walk of about 200 yards out front about 2:30.

She got to the kitchen about 11:00 June 8th. I told her I ate an omelet and she asked how you make an omelet. I made one for her. I suggested a walk about 12:30 and she asked about lunch. I reminded her she did not eat breakfast till about 11:00. We ate lunch after the walk. Lunch went very well. She can be so alert at times and then there are other times. She is much stronger than she was or she could not make the walk we make regularly. I thank our Lord for her improvement, but also wonder how much longer either of us has here. Oh well, at our ages how much longer can we expect? I am convinced that after more than forty one years together we belong together. Our life together has not been perfect, but it has been wonderful. I remember the old song "I don't know what the future holds, but I know Who holds the future." I started talking with her about things that happened while she was in the hospital and nursing home. She was responsive and we had about twenty minutes of two way conversation. We discussed many serious and very personal things. Then we had a very pleasant meal. After eating I replaced a burned out light bulb. She helped by handing me the bulb so I did not need to get off the ladder. It was more than two hours of the best time we have had in a long time. Do you say that does not sound like a big deal? From where she has been the last twenty two months or so it is wonderful to see her mind working so good for any period of time.

At 9:50 PM she said she had not made the bed. I helped her out of the chair and she walked to the bathroom. I made the bed. This has been a good day.

Neither of us got a good night's sleep the night of June 10th-11th. We got up at 4:30 AM because I have a seminar. She did dress on time and Bell helped her with breakfast after I left.

I decided to try something new for lunch. I asked her to go to the kitchen and see what we had and what she wanted for lunch. She spent about fifteen minutes in the kitchen and made no suggestions. Then I saw she was holding a can of white chicken in her hand. I said that was what we were having for lunch. I opened the can and told her to prepare it. I walked across the room. She made sandwiches and poured drinks without my help. Lunch was good, but dinner was not so good. Dinner sounds like a replay of the old routine.

At 8:00 PM I remembered we had not done the walk out front. I suggested it and she was ready. We made it with no difficulty except it was a little difficult for her to get down and up the drive. A year ago I never dreamed we would do that walk together. My faith was too weak.

Sunday morning she started to say the old "I can't" and I told her not to say that. I helped her start dressing and she was ready much quicker than I expected. We continue to read The Purpose Driven Life. She reads it out loud and I listen. I believe it is good for her to do the reading. We had a considerable discussion after reading it this afternoon.

She came home from the nursing home a year ago today, June 16th. Could this be called some kind of an anniversary?

When I suggested the walk out front she chose not to do it. After church she walked with me to where the car was parked. That was a considerable distance and up a rather steep incline. She had no trouble walking as I held her arm.

While I was preparing dinner she came to the kitchen and started crying. I took her to the bedroom and told her to come back when she quit crying. I also told her the bed was not made. She came back to the kitchen in a few minutes and was not crying as much. Later I went back and found she had made the bed. I blew it again. Dinner was not exactly a joyous affair. I told her what I was getting for desert and asked what she wanted. She did not reply. She finally got up and got fruit from the frig. Things were going quite well at bedtime.

June 21st started off about as usual. She went to the bank with me and then I went to the post office. She did not ask what I was mailing. That is not like her because she always wanted to know everything that is going on in our lives, and I believed she should. I did not tell her what I was mailing because I wanted to see if she would ask. In mid afternoon we read the final chapter of The Purpose Driven Life. We did the walk out front about 4:00. In spite of these things she was very low, and there was very little talk.

We went out for dinner June 25th and I ordered first because it was obvious she did not know what to order. I ordered a meal I knew she would like except one vegestable

I like but she does not. She asked for the same and I asked if she wanted that vegestable. She said no. It took a long time for her to choose. She is so much better, but I remember that wonderful wife who had such a brilliant mind.

We read the Sunday school lesson together. When we went to bed she was very low.

While we were eating dinner out I showed her a letter I had written to a local newspaper which was published in the letters to the editor. I asked if she saw where it came from. She said she did, but she made no comment.

When we were ready to go to church in the evening I told her I knew she could get out of the chair by herself if she wanted to. She got up without my help. I said I refuse to let her think of herself as an invalid.

We had breakfast together about 8:00 June 28th. After this wonderful start lunch was bad. Dinner went fairly well.

I told her June 30th I like to see her in a dress more often. She said she did not have a dress she could wear. I picked one of her nicer dresses and she put it on without a lot of resistance. After church I reminded her at least three people complemented her on her dress. She did not say a word.

She has made the bed several times recently. In order to let her feel she can do something I frequently leave the bed unmade just to see what she will do. At about 8:30 she said she had not made the bed. We made it together.

She reminded me of a friend who was injured in an accident. I called him and we had a nice three way conversation. After we hung up she and I had more conversation than we have had in a long time. It was near what could be called normal home life.

We had a good dinner in the frig that only needed to be warmed up. As I got it out she said she did not know how to prepare it. I told her to let me do it. I asked her to set the table and she did it. I asked if she wanted a tomato and lettuce salad and she said no. I fixed a salad in one bowl and she said that was too much for me. I said if she did not take some I would eat it all. She took very little of it. She seems to be afraid she will eat too much.

There is an art show downtown tonight between 5 and 9. When she got the card I asked if she wanted to go and she did not say. I asked again this afternoon and she did not answer. She picked up the card about 7:00. At 7:15 she came to the living room with the card in her hand. I asked what she was up to, and she did not answer. I thought she wanted to go to the art show, but did not want to push it. I finally asked if she wanted to go and she said she guessed so. She knew exactly which gallery the lady she wanted to see was in. She walked at least three tenths of a mile from where I parked to the gallery. She was not too tired when we got home. It was a good evening.

I tried to talk with her after we went to bed. I said I regret a lot of things I have done since she has been sick, such as loosing my temper and my language at times. I said I have been under a lot of pressure, but I take full responsibility. I asked if she could understand. She said yes to everything I asked, but she said nothing else. She would not say anything even when I said her not talking with me makes me feel like I am living alone, even when we are in the same house.

We had a special July 4th service and dinner at the church and got home about 6:30. About 8:00 we sat on the back porch awhile where we had a nice conversation. She did not have such a sad look. Then I went to sleep in the chair. When I woke she was in the bathroom. She said she called me and I did not respond.

I decided to see a new doctor for myself and insisted she see him too. She was not happy about this. By the time dinner was over I was crying more than she was.

When we woke July 7th she said she knew I would think she was crazy, but she did not know what to put on.

She said she wanted to help. I asked what she wanted to help with and she said help with getting dinner. It was about time to get dinner. We went to the kitchen. I showed her every little detail. As we ate I said it seems more like a meal she cooked. She said she did this recently. I did not say it to her, but that sounds like the dementia. There was considerable two way talk. Could this be a turning point? I really do not know. I have done so many things that even I question. Then I try to justify my actions. There are some things I cannot explain.

When I returned from the men's breakfast about 9:10 July 9th she was in the bathroom, but not dressed. With little help from me she was in the kitchen about 9:50. For dinner I tried to do a replay of last night and asked her to do more. It went fairly well, but not as good as last night.

We were awake at 5:00 AM July 10th and she said happy birthday. I said I appreciated that. We woke again about 7:00 and she was ready to eat about 9:10 with practically no help from me. When she came out I told her she could get her own breakfast, or I would help her. She did most of it. I tell her, and I really believe, the more she can do for herself the more confidence it gives her. After eating she did the back porch routine and we sat on the back porch awhile. We did the walk out front about 11:15.

Sunday, July 11th, she came to the living room about 7:50 and said she did not put on a slip because she did not have one. I took her back to the bedroom and found a slip where they are normally kept. She put it on. We drove downtown to eat. On the way way home she started some small talk three times. When we got home we both went to sleep in the chairs. When we woke she spoke in a very normal voice and I told her that was great.

July 13th I asked her to mix a can of orange juice that I had thawed out. She did it after I opened the can. In midafternoon she indicated she wanted to get out of the chair. I helped her up and we did the walk out front.

I went to the bedroom about midafternoon and saw the bed had been made. I said I did not remember making it. She said "I made it". Dinner at home went good and there was some talk.

Lunch and dinner went Ok the next day. She said what she needed was less food. I said I continue to be cooncerned about the weight she has lost.

We did the walk out front. We ate dinner out and met friends who invited us to join them. Then at home we watched gospel music on TV.

She woke me July 18th and said it was 6:10. That was about an hour earlier than we needed to get up. It was not difficult to get her up, but it did take some encouraging. After I walked out she called me and said she made a mistake by putting on panty hose. I said that could be changed, but she did not do it. I picked a slip and dress which she put on quicker than I expected. She would not say what she wanted for breakfast. I suggested cereal, bacon and egg, or an omelet. She asked how to make an omelet. We ate omelets. In the afternoon I suggested doing the walk out front and she said no. Sundays we usually leave about 6:05 for the evening service. At 5:45 she said she was readdy. I said it was too early to leave. She was ready to do the walk.

We woke at 6:50 July 19th and she did not say a word. I got up at 7:25 and asked if she wanted to get up and eat with me. She said "I don't know". I went back about 8:45 and set a glass of orange juice in her bath room. I told her it was there when she wanted to get up and get it. She got to the kitchen about 10:00. When she finished eating I asked if she wanted more. She said "I certainly do not". She is always afraid she will eat too much.

We left about 7:45 AM for her colonscopy exam. The doctor said he saw nothing to be alarmed about. After the recovery room we went to a buffet where she ate a good meal.

She said she did not know what to prepare for lunch. I told her to go to the kitchen, see what was there, and make a choice. She got off the chair with no help from me, went to the kitchen, and made a choice. She chose a can which I opened for her. My plan was to see what she could and would do and it worked. After eating she asked me to clean the dishes and put them in the dishwasher. I was happy to do that. I tried the same plan for dinner, but it did not work.

As we were watching gospel music on TV I said something about what I would like to see again as compared to things in our past livess together. She smiled like I had not seen her smile in a long time. Soon after that she smiled again about the same. That was a wonderful few seconds.

She dressed rather quickly Sunday, July 25th, and put on one of her nicest dresses.

She woke me about 5:00 the next morning. I got up about 6:30. She was sobbing. I set a glass of orange juice on the bathroom sink about 8:30 and told her she could get it when she got up. I walked out again. Lunch was another rough time.

The next day she dressed without help from me. Lunch was OK, and we did the walk out front about 4:30. As I started to get dinner I said I had to empty the dish washed. She said she did that while I was at the grocery. I mentioned a couple who had moved from our area. I asked if we had not heard they were dead. She said she remembered hearing the lady was dead, but did not remember about him. She said that in a very normal voice.

She seemed to be in fair shape at 7:15 July 31st. I took her orange juice in about 9:00 and encouraged her to get up. I told her she needed something to eat. She was ready about 10:00. She did several things to help get lunch. I told her I am working hard to get her well. I said I am a hard task master. She said "you're a task master all right". That sounded good to me. She said something.

When we woke about 7:00 Aug 3rd we had a very nice two way convesstion. I got up about 7:30 and when I went back about 8:30 it was the same old routine. She was in the kitchen when we prepared dinner and it was one of the best meals we have had recently.

She called me at 8:45 Aug 4th. I had to force her to let me start dressing her. She was in the kitchen ready to eat at 9:45. She talked a little. Lunch was pleasant and we did the walk out front about 2:30. She needed help to get out of the chair at bed time.

We had a pitch in dinner at the home of some friends. While eating the men sat at one table and the ladies at another. When we got home I asked what the ladies talked about. She told me nothing. I told her some of the things we discussed includiddng one man that was going to Africa to hunt big game. Then I told her the story about the big game hunter. I said something he disagreed with ate him.

I do not remember when I had heard her laugh so much. This has been a good day.

We saw her regular physician. He was quite pleased with her condition and did not mention her taking any more medication.

August 8th started with her dressing quicker and with no help from me. We had considerable conversation when we woke Aug 9th. We did the walk out front about 4:00, and dinner went well. After dinner she walked toward the bathroom and I thought she was gone a long time. I went in and found her making the bed.

She was quite pleasant when she woke Aug 10th, but then said she did not know what to put on. She got to the kitchen about 9:30 and quicker than usual she told me what she wanted to eat.

I am learning that unless there is a special need to get her up earlier it is better to let her do her own thing and get up when she wants to. Then there is also the fact she needs breakfast before lunch time. What do I do?

She called me about an hour after I got up Aug 18th because she was having trouble dressing. I helped her start dressing. She put on a nice dress. Later she reminded me that was the day of the ladies' luncheon.

She got up in time to have breakfast with me Aug 19th.

When I got back from the men's breakfast Aug 20th about 9:00 I did not insist she get up till 10:30. She finished breakfast about 11:30 and asked about lunch at 12:50. We went to the grocery about 4:30 and she made some good suggestions. We went downtown and she had less trouble choosing some things she needed.

When we woke Aug 21st I told her I had a wonderful dream last night. I really wanted to talk with her about it. She did not reply. Later in the day I got her to the computer and showed her what I had written about the dream. She showed me some corrections I should make, but never said a word about what I really wanted to talk about.

After eating dinner Aug 23rd I said something about taking a drive where we could see the sunset. Several minutes later she asked where we could go to see the sunset. We drove to a nearby park and sat on a walk bridge to watch the stream. It was just a walk in the park, but we enjoyed it.

Some time ago I loaned my notes about her case to a friend. He read them and made a very helpful analysis for me. I had asked her before if she wanted to read his analysis, and she made no comment. Today I asked her to read the first page and more if she wanted to. She read all of it and made some very interesting comments. Lunch at home was nice, and we did the walk out front.

While I was getting dinner she cried so much I had to take her out of the kitchen. That is the first time I have had to do that in two weeks or more. In about five minutes she went back to the kitchen and set the table. She cried very little. Dinner and the evening went quite well.

August 26th, 2004 I mentioned a particular chicken and rice recipe she made before her illness which I loved. I showed her a recipe a friend had written for me which I thought was hers. She told me whose recipe that was and she told me how to make hers, including the temperature to set the oven. We went to the store and got the ingredients to make it. I wrote this recipe down so we could enjoy it in the future.

August 29th she told me she did not know if she had told me or not, but she had to go to the hospital when she was in school. I had heard nothing about this before. She could not remember the details, but it appears she was about twelve or thirteen years old. She could not remember what her trouble was or how long she was in the hospital. She seemed to think she could have been in the hospital for months. She could remember her mother visiting her, but could not remember her father or half brother visiting her. I said it was interesting to me she could not remember her father visiting her because she had told me earlier she could remember going to the viewing for her father, but could not remember going to his funeral. I asked if she ever had problems with her father or her brother. She said she did not. I told her this conversation was very interesting to me, and could possibility be helpful in her recovery.

We picked up some clothes she had altered. When we got to the bedroom she said she did not know what to do. I said it was like trying on a new dress she was buying.

When we woke August 31st she was more like she was years ago than I had seen in a long time. We had considerable pleasant conversation.

The next day she seemed to be in good spirits when she woke, but then started whimpering. She got to the kitchen for breakfast about 11:00.

When I went back September 2nd she said she did not know what to put on. I told her the first thing to put on was a smile, and then she could see her clothes. I went back at 9:25. She had just gotten out of bed and was in tears.

She started toward the bedroom about 8:30 PM September 3rd and said the bed had not been made. We made it together.

She got to the kitchen just after 12:00 noon September 4th. We ate lunch about 1:30 and then went to the grocery. We woke earlier Sunday, September 5th. She called me at 7:45 and needed help with the zipper which was on the back of her dress. We had a church picnic dinner at 5:00.

She did most of the work preparing the chicken and rice dish she remembered recently.

September 7th was a very good day. We went downtown in the afternoon. The evening was quiet and after we went to bed we had considerable conversation.

She seemed much better when she woke September 14th, but was in tears when I got up. She was in the kitchen before 10:00. We did the walk out front. We continue to have some two way conversation. I would not call it normal, but it is better than it was two or three months ago. She set the table and dinner went quite well.

I insisted she get up earlier September 18th because I needed to go out. She finished breakfast about 10:30 and she was very silent. We ate dinner out. The turkey and dressisng was delicious, but she said she could not eat all that was on her plate. As we went to bed I said something stupid and she laughed out loud.

I left at 9:25 Monday to go to a funeral. She did not want to go. When I got back at 11:20 she was in bed, and I insisted she get up. When she finally decided what she wanted to eat she put bacon and egg in the frying pan. Dinner at home went quite well and there was some conversation in the evening.

I insisted she get up at 9:00 AM September 21st and then I walked out. When I went back she said something about not knowing what to do. I did nothing to help her dress, and she came out ready to eat at 11:00. Lunch and dinner at home went OK. We did the walk out front about 4:40.

She has talked more the last two months or so. I am not saying our conversations are normal, because they are so short. I am saying things are better than they were.

About dinner time September 27th she reminded me of a meeting we should go to which started at 6:30. I had forgotten it. We were late, but we went.

She called me at 10:00 September 30th because she was having trouble dressisng. I went back and helped her get started, and then walked out. She finished eating about 10:30 and then washed her dishes. Lunch at home was OK, and we did the walk out front. Dinner at home went well, and then we watched the presendital debate.

I planned to cook chicken chow mein for dinner. When I mentioned it to her she said she did not know how to cook it. When I put it on the two plates she said that was too much, but she ate her part of it. That has happened before.

I told her I had an omelet for breakfast October 2nd and she asked how I made it. She decided she wanted the same. It was about 60 degrees outside. She went to the bike and said it was cold out there. I told her to get on the bike and shake a leg and she would warm up. She did not seem to agree, but she did the bike ride. We did the walk out front in the afternoon.

Things were not too different when we got up October 5th or for lunch. We did the walk out front in the afternoon. Dinner did not go good. We watched the vice presidential debates, and then the 700 Club. When we went to bed she seemed to feel better than I did.

She called me about 9:00 October 6th because she needed help dressing. I helped her start and then walked out. She got to the kitchen about 10:00. I told her I would do anything I could do for her, but I thought it was good for her to do anything she could. She looked around awhile and then prepared cereal for herself. We did the outside walk in the afternoon and went to the church dinner and prayer meeting.

She was ready to eat at 8:30 October 8th and we had breakfast together. It was a better than usual day.

October 11th I suggested she call her friend Ruth about the problem she had in 1960. At 8:00 PM she told me it was 9:00 where Ruth lived. That told me she wanted to make the call. She talked with Ruth more than I thought she would. Ruth could tell us nothing I believe is important. Ruth believes my thinking something is buried in her mind is not important. I believe it is very important. She was calm when we went to bed.

It amazes me that she has made so much improvement. We now have some communication, but it is always so short. I get so lonely when we can make no plans for the future, and have communications so seldom.

Sunday, October 17th started out about as usual except she got to the kitchen earlier than usual. We went to the quarterly board meeting at Potter's Clay. About 10:00 PM she said she did not know what to do to get organized. We went to bed a little before 11:00 and lay there and talked for about an hour. That was wonderful. When she woke the next morning it was a totally different story.

I went to the grocery soon after getting up October 20th. When I got back she was eating breakfast. I took her to the ladies' luncheon and we did the walk out front.

October 21st when she said she did not know what to put on I told her to put on a smile. I wanted to go to a certain meeting at 6:30 PM. She would not say whether she wanted to go till we finished eating just befor 6:00. We went. We had more than the usual talk in the evening. The next day went quite well, and there was considerable conversation in the evening.

Sunday I suggested she wear her new outfit which I like. I helped her start dressing and then walked out. She put on the same dress she had worn the last three times we went to anything she would dress up for. When we got home I stopped out front and we did the outside walk without walking up or down the steep drive.

When I started to eat October 25th I could not find some syrup I purchased a few days ago, and I decided she must have put it away. She got up and found it with no trouble.

It was almost 12:00 noon when she ate breakfast October 26th and even at that time she ate less than she usually eats for breakfast. She did the back porch routine. Lunch and dinner at home were very well. She was calm at bed time. After she finally got out of bed it has been a very good day.

October 27th was a fairly good day.

I took her orange juice in at 8:30 October 30th and encouraged her to get up. Prior to my helping her start dressing she said something about not knowing what to put on. Then she said she did not have anything to put on her legs. I showed her where her hose was in the dresser. I looked in about 10:00 and she was in the kitchen. She did her bike ride.

Sunday, October 31, I suggested she wear something different because she had worn the same thing so often lately. She dressed herself in a different outfit and was in the kitchen rather quickly.

She talked quite a bit when we woke November 1st. She called me about 8:35. She was near tears and needed help dressing.

She was in good shape when we woke November 2nd. I went back after I ate and she was in bad shape. I practically forced her to let me put her underclothes on her, and then I walked out. She finished dressing. We watched the election reports on TV that night.

The next day I said I did nothing to help her dress and she made no comment. We did the outside walk and the day went quite well.

While I was working in the yard November 6th she called me and said she could not find a certain part of the blender in the dish washer as she was taking the dishes out of the washer. The piece was clear plastic and I had put it where it would be easy to overlook. I found it for her. She called me about 7:55 AM November 8th and her voice sounded like something tragic had happened. I rushed to her in the bedroom. She showed me her ring had broken. It looked like something in the clasp that holds it together had broken. I told her the jeweler could repair it. Since I had a cold I laid down after lunch and took a nap. When I woke she was unloading the dish washer.

When she got up November 10th and said something about not knowing what to put on I made some remark and she slapped me on the shoulder. I laughed at her and walked out. While she was eating breakfast I walked out. When I went back she was washsing her dishes.

About 5:00 PM November 11th she said something about not knowing what to wear to the ladies' meeting which started at 7:00. I encouraged her to change. I prepared dinner while she was changing. When she got back to the kitchen she set the table. I took her to the meeting.

When I got back from the men's breakfast about 9:15 she said she had not had anything to eat. That was something new. We went to Wal Mart after lunch and she bought some hose but was just not able to choose other things she needed. After dinner I said this had been a good day and she said she guessed it had been.

She dressed with no help from me November 13th. As we were eating November 14th she said I had gained weight because my jacketed looked tighter.

While she was eating breakfast November 15th she reminded me a friend had invited her to play scrabble with her today, and we were to call her this morning. I suggested she make the call and much to my pleasant surprise she did.

We had a nice conversation when we woke November 18th. When I took her orange juice in about 8:30 she was near tears.

Sunday morning started with her saying she did not know what to wear. I mentioned three or four outfits and walked out. She dressed rather quickly with no help from me. I told her I was eating a waffle and she said she wanted the same. Breakfast went good.

The next day she came to the office room about 11:30 and told me she put the laundry in the dryer. I had forgotten it.

I talk with her occasionally about the notes I am writing. I showed her some notes Marie had given me about certain changes she thought should be made in my notes. Helen studied this for some time and asked some questions.

She talked quite a bit when we woke November 25th. Just after eating breakfast she asked if I had put the laundry in the dryer. I had not. We had Thanksgiving dinner with friends at their home.

She got up before I did November 26th and there was some talk before she got up. We had breakfast together. She made the bed by herself about 10:30.

We did the walk out front about 4:00. In the late afternoon she asked what we were having for dinner. She does not do that often.

She seemed to be in a better mood when she woke November 27th. When I took her orange juice in about 8:30 she was sobbing. She dressed with no help from me and got to the kitchen at 9:25. I just sat and watched her get her breakfast. Lunch went OK and we did the walk out front. While we were walking I said it was a little chilly. She said "it is more than a little chilly". It was about 60. I showed her something that came in the E-mail. She said she had seen that before. OH that dementia.

When she woke November 29th her voice was as normal as I ever heard it—even before her illness. She spoke very little after that, but her voice continued to be normal. Then in about half an hour she started sobbing. Just before bedtime we had considerable conversation about some very enjoyable times in the past. I was on Cloud 9. When I got to the bedroom she was crying.

She finished breakfast about 10:30 December 3rd and about 12:00 she asked me to help her make the bed. We had Christmas dinner with two Sunday school classes. When she started to bed she got out of the chair with no help from me.

When I started to get lunch December 4th she reminded me we were out of bread so we ate lunch out.

She said she was ready to eat about 10:00 December 6th. I told her to help herself, and then I went to her immediately. She did most of the work getting her breakfast.

She fried her own bacon and egg December 7th. We had some normal talk while she was eating.

She woke me at 5:00 the next morning when she turned on the light to see what time it was. She talked some. I woke again about 6:00 and she talked some more. Then she started sobbing. She said she did not know what to put on. As I walked out I said "So what's new?." With my help she prepared the food for the church dinner tonight.

I did not offer to help her dress December 9th. She called at 9:55 and said she was ready to eat. I told her the two choices for lunch at home or we could go out. Fifteen minutes later she said she wanted to go out, and even told me where she wanted to go.

December 10th she told me it was time to get up if I wanted to go to the men's breakfast. I went to the grocery after breakfast December 11th. I told her I expected her to be dressed when I got back. When I got back she was not only dressed, but almost finished eating breakfast. I started working in the yard at 11:00 and she called at 12:45 and asked when I wanted lunch. Lunch was not really pleasant, but dinner was nice. When we went to bed about 10:30 we talked about some very serious things. She said something happened before our marriage, but she could not remember what it was. I said when we are able to talk about it she will get better, or well. We decided to go to sleep about 12:30. I slept some. She said she did not sleep any. I have told her many times in the past, as a joke, we don't dare talk about any big deals or it will keep her from sleeping. I worked in the yard some December 13th. When I went back she said a friend had called and told me what the call was about. She very rarely takes a phone call.

When we woke Sunday, December 19th, she was in better shape. She got up and dressed without my help much quicker than usual. She even told me what she wanted to eat much quicker than usual.

She dressed with no help from me December 21st and she put the bacon and egg in the frying pan. She did the back porch routine.

When we woke December 24th she said good morning and then did not say another word. She sobbed a big part of the time till I got up. I ate, shoveled snow off the drive, and then went to the bedroom about 10:00. I jerked the cover off her and told her to get up. She did not like that, but she got up. I started to the living room about 5:25 PM and saw her coming toward the office. She wore a smile like I had not seen in a long time, and I told her I liked that. We had a very pleasant dinner, and during the evening there was more communication than we usually have.

Can this be Christmas day? We had looked forward to the Christmas eve service last night, but it was cancelled because of the weather. I know we look forward to His coming again. This is the third Christmas since Helen got sick. We ate dinner downtown. We had a safe trip even though we saw several weather related accidents.

We had a New Year's Eve party at the church which started at 6:00 with a pot luck dinner. She came to the kitchen about 8:30 January 1st, 2005 while I was eating. She had dressed with no help from me.

She did the usual things to help me get lunch January 3rd. Dinner went well. Some time after 7:00 we finished going through the mail which came late. The mail included Christmas letters from two ladies who were friends of hers. We had at least an hour of two way conversation which was great. We had more conversation just after we turned off the TV at 11:00.

She dressed quicker than usual January 4th and got to the kitchen just as I finished eating. I asked what she wanted to eat and she said "a waffle I guess". I said I wished she would be postive about something. She put the batter on the waffle iron and prepared her own breakfast.

When it was about time to get dinner January 7th I told her to go to the kitchen, see what was available, and tell me what she wanted. Later she said it was 5:30. I said she had not told me what she wanted for dinner. I prepared dinner, and she set the table and put food on the plates. Dinner was good even though there was almost no talk.

She woke me Sunday January 9th at 6:00 and said she had not slept any. We got up about 7:00 and I had to dress her. In the afternoon I slept some in the chair, and she said she guessed she slept some. She talked some and even gave me two or three nice smiles. There was a limited amount of conversation in the evening.

When I got up January 11th I told her a couple of things I needed to do and said when I get back I hope she is dressed. When I got back about 9:30 she was dressed and in the kitchen preparing her breakfast. Lunch and dinner at home went OK.

I took her to a ladies' brunch which started at 10:15. When we got back it was about 1:00. She said she did not want anything more to eat. When my lunch was ready she decided she did want to eat. I was happy that she wanted to eat again because she always seems to fear she will eat too much. We had dinner at the church. We were in the kitchen about 9:35 doing a small detail. I asked what she wanted to eat and she said more food was what she did not need. She talked more today and it was in a normal tone.

She woke me at 5:00 AM January 15th and told me I forgot to do the laundry last night. I went back to sleep. I went back at 8:30 and told her it was time to get up. She got to the kitchen about 10:00 and did most of the work preparing her ham and egg breakfast. Then the back porch routine. Lunch and dinner at home went OK.

She was in much better shape when we woke January 16th. I helped her start dressisng and she finished quicker than usual. There was some talk before church and after we got home. After the evening service I got her to go to the computer to look at some of the notes I am preparing about her case for a short review I am sending to Dr Josef. She seemed to read the first page and she found a typo. She said it was not the way she remembered it. I am not sure of the wisdom of this, but I would like to get her approval—especially if any of it is ever published. It has been a better day.

January 17th I asked her to come to the computer to see my new web site. She watched it with considerable interest.

She seemed to be in fair shape when we woke January 20th, but was sobbing in a few minutes. I went to the bathroom and she thought I had left the house. She called and asked me to bring her orange juice. She got to the kitchen about 9:45 and finally decided she wanted bacon and egg which I prepared. She was so low at lunch time. It was another of those cold silence times. Dinner was some better and there was a limited amount of two way conversation in the evening.

Last night I said I would like for her to get a new pair of dress shoes because the pair she has been wearing hurt her feet. She has not been able to choose what she needs. About 5:30 she asked what we were going to do. I asked what she meant. She said I mentioned going downtown. She said where she would like to eat as we were driving downtown. We got her shoes. There was more than the usual two way conversation this evening.

When we woke January 22nd she said I did not pick up the mail yesterday. She was right. She also said the microwave was not working. I thought she was wrong, but then remembered the power went off yesterday. Then I made the adjustments for the microwave.

I helped her start dressing January 27th and she finished rather quickly. We made the bed after she ate, and she did the back porch routine. She was very low at lunch time, and I was so low I was near tears. Dinner was better. She set the table and put the food on the plates. After we ate I started putting things in the trash for tomorrow's pick up and, without a word from me, she washed the dishes.

When I got back from the men's breakfast about ten minutes later than uusual she met me in the living room and said she thought she heard me come in earlier. She was not dressed but had her coat on. Lunch was not exciting, but there were no real problems. Dinner at home went very well.

When she called January 29th and said she did not know what to put on I told her the first thing to put on was a smile. I helped her start dressing and then walked out. She finished and was in the kitchan before 9:00. In the evening I brought up the idea of possibly having these notes published. I said we have watched many people's personal stories on the 700 Club. We agreed we do not condem them. She never said she approved or disapproved of the idea. When we shut off the TV I said she looked like she was thinking. She did not reply.

She got up on her own January 31st and was ready to eat before 9:00. She did most of the work preparing her breakfast. After eating she did the bike ride and we made the bed.

When I took the dishes out of the dishwasher in midafternoon February 1st she noticed we needed jet dry for the dishwasher. We went to the store to get jet dry and something else I had forgotten. I did this more to pacify her than for the immediate need. When we got to the store she went one way to get one product and I went the other way to get the other. Just think. A doctor told me she would die more than two years ago.

Something on TV brought back memories of friends years ago. This led to considerable two way conversation.

When we woke February 8th she was sobbing and did not say a word to me.

Again, when we woke February 10th she was sobbing and did not say a word. When I went back at 9:15 she was dressed and ready to go to the kitchen. By looking at the kitchen she could see I ate a waffle. Much quicker than usual she said she wanted a waffle. When I started preparing dinner I received a phone call she thought would last awhile. She indicated I should cut it short, and later reminded me she has a ladies' meeting at 7:00. After the meeting she told me more about it than any meeting since she has been sick. I told her I appreciate that.

When we woke February 14th she did not say a word. When I took her orange juice in about 8:00 I said she could not stay in bed till noon. She was sitting on the side of the bed about 8:40, and I suggested she get up. It was a major job getting her started dressing. The last two days I mentioned going out for a valentine dinner tonight and she never said yes or no. I mentioned it again today. At about 4:30 she told me where she wanted to go.

When we woke February 16th she seemed to be in good shape, but then started sobbing. She said she did not know what to put on, and then reminded me it was the day of the ladies' luncheon. When she got to the kitchen she had slacks on. She never wears slacks to the luncheon. After she ate I insisted she put on better clothes and she said she did not have anything else. She finally put on a dress and I took her to the luncheon. Dinner was pot luck at the church. She was in good shape at bed time.

About dinner time February 18th I asked what she wanted to do for dinner. Fifteen minutes later she had not replied. Then she went to the bedroom and got her coat. She asked if we were going out. We ate out.

We went to the grocery in the afternoon of February 19th and she made several good suggestions. Dinner at home went well. I mentioned apple pie and ice cream. Several minutes later she said she wanted a small piece of pie and ice cream. I said she always says I serve too much, so I told her to cut the size of pie she wanted. She did it. After eating we read tomorrow's Sunday school lesson and then watched gospel music on TV. The Gaither program was different and Helen laughed a lot. It has been a much better day.

She did not say much when we woke February 22nd. I helped her start dressing and she finished. There was nothing unusual about the day.

She finished breakfast about 9:30 February 23rd. She was very low at lunch and started crying. I picked up my plate and told her I was going to the other room if she did not quit crying. She stopped crying immediately and I stayed with her.

She talked some before I got up February 24th. She asked if I had put the laundry in the dryer and I had forgotten it. I told her I appreciated her reminding me. She called me later and I helped her start dressing.

She asked how many men were at the men's breakfast. When I named them she asked if Walt was not the one who is not a member or our church. She was right. She knows what is going on, but is just not able to do much on her own.

She talked a little when we woke February 26th. She called me about 9:00 and I helped her start dressing. There was no big difference the remainder of the day.

After eating out February 27th I turned toward Hot Springs. She asked where we were going. I told her we were going to the springs to get water. I did not tell her before because I wanted to see if she would say anything to me. I went to sleep in the chair about 10:00 PM and she woke me just before 11:00. She said she forgot to turn on the 700 Club. I said I do not recommend that because it is not on Sundays. She laughed out loud. I love to hear those infrequent laughs.

Dinner at home February 28th went well and I ran the dishwasher after we ate. I was reading about 9:00 PM and she told me it was time to empty the dishwasher. I told her I was reading and if she wanted the dishwasher emptied to get off her rear and do it. That was not the way I should have handled it, but she got up and emptied the dishwasher. She said she did not know where to put certain things. I showed her where they go and she did the job.

She said she did not know what to do when she got up March 1st. She was dressed at 9:00 with no help from me, and she did most of the work in frying bacon and egg.

We went to a new doctor March 2nd that, due to my insistasnce, she had seen once or twice before. The main reason I insisted on her going was she had a sore on her leg that looked serious to me. He prescribed a cream for that and recommended she go on Zoloft.

When we woke the next day we had a limited amount of conversation. I looked for the Zoloft which I wanted her to take last night, but did not see it. She showed me where it was. Looking at the card it was obvious she had taken it. She started the old story about having nothing to wear. I disputed that, helped her start dressing, and walked out. She finished dressing and went to the kitchen before 9:00. She made the bed without my help. We went to the grocery in the evening. She was very slow, but she made some suggestions, and she read the instructions on several things she was considering buying. She was not the excellent shopper she was years ago but it looked like the Helen of years ago was trying to come back. The evening at home went quite well with nothing too different.

She did not say what she wanted to eat March 5th but she stood by the waffle iron. I asked if she wanted a waffle and she said yes. Together we prepared it. Then she did the back porch routine.

When we woke the next morning I said something about it being Monday. She told me it was Sunday and she was right.

She was sobbing when she woke March 8th and did not speak to me even when I mentioned it was her birthday. When she got to the kitchen a little before 9:00 I just sat and watched as she got her breakfast. When she put bread in the toaster she asked me to butter it for her. I said that was the first word she had spoken to me this morning. She said she did not realize that. We went to the grocery in the afternoon. On the way home I said she had not told me where she wanted to go for her birthday dinner, and if she did not tell me I would cook dinner and say no more about it. She said nothing. At about 5:30 she told me where she wanted to go and we went there.

March 9th was not too different except we put together the dish we took to the church dinner and she did most of that.

I helped her start dressing Sunday, March 13th, and then I walked out. She finished dressing quicker than usual and breakfast was pleasant. When we got to the car in the attached garage I noticed she did not have a coat on, not even a sweater. It was about fifty degrees. I asked which coat she wanted, and I went back and got it. When we started to leave for the evening service she asked where her coat was. I got it for her. As I was standing behind her putting her coat on her she fell backwards. She would have hit the floor if I had not been there. I caught her, so there was no injury.

She was in the kitchen about 8:00 the next morning with no help from me.

She called about 8:30 March 16th because she was having trouble dressisng. I helped her start and then walked out. After a normal morning I took her to the monthly ladies' luncheon. We had dinner at the church.

She called me at 7:45 March 17th to call my attention to two school busses stopped in fromnt of our house. It appeared one had mechanical trouble and the other came out to get the school children. I went back at 9:05 and helped her start dressing. I was walking across the room with my back to her. As I looked back I saw she had fallen and her hand hit the coffee table which prevented her hitting the floor. There was no injury, but it scared me. After eating dinner I asked if she wanted to go to the grocery with me. After a long hesitation she got her coat. When we got home she put the groceries away. When we started to bed she reminded me tomorrow is garbage pick up day. I had forgotten to put it out.

We were awake about 6:00 March 19th and she was talking very little. I looked in at 9:00 and she was well on her way dressing, and I had done nothing to help her. She finished eating about 9:45 and did the back porch routine. There was some talk as she was eating. Lunch and dinner at home went quite well.

Getting her started March 21st was not too bad. She finished breakfast about 10:00. Lunch at 1:00 was not good. While preparing dinner I felt she was looking at what I was doing in a critical way. Maybe she was grieving because she was not able to do it. When she cannot talk with me how can I tell? I broke down again.

About 5:00 PM March 22nd she told me her eye was hurting. From what she told me I thought she had something in it, and she said it started about 1:45. We went to the ER. It was an infection.

At about 8:15 PM March 24th I suggested a game of UpWords. She acted like she wanted to get out of the chair and I helped her. She just stood there and I did nothing except watch her. About fifteen minutes later she said something to the effect we should play. She played a fairly good game. One time when I made a suggestion she said she did not know what had happened to her mind. I said we know she has problems, but her mind is getting better.

There was nothing too different about March 25th except we went to the Good Friday service at 3:00.

Both of us were awake about 6:00 March 28th and she talked very normally. I was thrilled.

She was sobbing at 7:45. It amazes me how much either of us can change in such a short time. I brought up the question of where we would have been if we had given up in the early part of her illness. I said I believe only our Lord has the power to keep us here, but I believe we have some responsibility. We were in agreement. I said I have seen her smile more today than in a long time—and that was true. She seemed surprised at that.

Someone asked me what the most difficult part of this is. It is the lack of communication. Can you imagine what it is like to live with someone you have loved so long and have no communications, and make no plans for the future? Yes, she is so much better than she was a year ago, but there continues to be so little communication. In the late evening she said there was something she could not remember. It appeared to be something she wanted to talk with me about. In a few minutes she said something about someone we had lived near in Indianapolis. Then she mentioned the lady had trouble with her leg. That gave me the clue it was the lady who lived near our present house. We had considerable conversation about this.

Late in the day April 1st I mentioned going after spring water which we use for cooking and drinking. After dinner she asked if we were going after water. We went. When we got back she reminded me I had not brought in the mail. Then she asked about a minor problem I had with my hand. How do you explain it? She is so alert to so many things, and then when I ask such simple questions she cannot respond.

After we ate dinner April 5th I decided to try something new. I took the dishes to the sink and sat down again. After several minutes she asked if I wanted anything else. I said yes and gave her three choices for desert. She finally said she wanted ice cream. Then I said I would flip with her to see who washes the dishes. I said heads I win and tails you lose. She said that means she loses either way. I said "sure". She got up and went to the sink. I told her I would do it, but she stayed at the sink. She started and I finished the job.

I insisted she get up about 9:00 April 8th when I got back from the men's breakfast. She was ready to eat at

10:00 and I had not helped her. Two men from Terminix came to inspect the damage done by the need for a new roof.

Then two roofers came to give bids. Prior to her illness she would have been with me helping make decisions. She had nothing to say. She seemed to understand what I was thinking, but had no ideas.

We normally park at the back of the church for Sunday school. After church we can walk up the ramp, walk up thirteen steps, or I can bring the car down to pick her up at the front. She walked up the thirteen steps today as she has done for several weeks. I always walk close behind her just in case. This seems like such an ordinary thing but when you have been where she has been, and get where you can do that———.

There was considerable small talk when we woke April 11th. She was sobbing when I took her orange juice in at 7:45. She was ready to eat at 10:00 with no help from me.

I looked in about 8:00 April 13th and she was standing by her closet. I helped her start dressing about ten mindutes later. I reminded her we were going out and asked if she did not want to wear a dress instead of slacks. She did not reply. I looked in at 8:35 and she was holding her hose as if she were ready to put them on. Five minutes later she was sitting on a chair putting on her hose. It is unbelievable to me that this brilliant lady who was such a wonderful wife for all those years can be in this condition. A client came in at 9:05 and when he left at 9:30 she was in the kitchen. When I got to the kitchen she had prepared her cereal and was preparing her toast. We attended the church dinner and service. One man told me how much better she seems. He said he had watched her as she went through the bufet line, and she seemed so much better.

The next morning about 9:30 I was on the phone talking with IRS about some very technical information when I heard her call me. It is not unusual for her to call me when she gets up, so I did not go in for a minute or two. When I went in I saw she had fallen and was sitting on the floor at the entrance of her closet. She had fallen on carpet and was not hurt. I quickly told the IRS lady what happened and helped her up. After helping her I went back to the phone call.

I suggested April 16th that we listen to a tape by Dr Paul Meyer which I received a few days before. His subject was the causes of depression and treatment at his clinic. She listened, but had nothing to say when I asked questions. She was in tears. This reinforced my belief she is grieving about something that happened before our marriage. What can I do except thank our Lord for the thirty nine and a half wonderful years we had before she got sick?

She dressed April 19th with no help from me and was ready to eat at 8:30.

When she got to the kitchen April 21st she saw the waffle iron out and asked if I had a waffle. I said I did and asked if she wanted one. She did not answer but plugged in the waffle iron. Together we prepared a waffle and bacon for her. She did the back porch routine and we sat on the back porch awhile. When dinner was ready I asked her to put the food on the plates. It was no surprise she put about half the vegetables on the plates. I put the remainder of one vegetable on the plates, and told her I need a full meal. This is not unusual. Both of us ate what was on the plates. She seems to fear eating too much.

For some time I have noticed a tightness in my chest at times. I felt this after I went to bed. I started swinging my arms which I will call exercising. This seemed to reduce the tightness. She had no idea why I was doing that and thought I was just acting silly. She laughed at me. It was good to see her laugh. I did not tell her why I did it.

I asked April 26th when she would finish the medicine the new doctor gave her. She said she finished it several days ago and did not know she was to take it after the sample he gave her. We had the prescription filled. I should have watched this closer. After dinner I suggested going for a drive since it was such a nice spring day. She did not reply. About fifteen minutes later she began moving in her chair and said something about going. We went.

She was sobbing when I woke April 28th and reminded me I said I wanted to wash the sheets today. With no encouragement from me she got up at 7:25.

She came out at 10:50 April 29th and said she was ready for breakfast.

Jokingly, I said she should have breakfast every day. While we were eating lunch I suggested we listen to a tape by Dr Paul Meyer which we had heard once before. She agreed to listen to it. I brought out the notes I had written December 11th, 2004 when she said something happened prior to our marriage which was not clear in her memory. She read my notes but would not discuss the subject. I am convinced something happened, but I do not know what. I tried again to convince her I would understand if she would discuss it with me. All she would say was "I don't know".

She talked a little when she woke the next morning.

Sunday night, May 1st, she told me in a very normal voice she needed to buy some new clothes. I told her I agreed. She has not been able to choose anything, and I am not good at choosing for her. The next day she was not able to choose anything.

There was some talk when she woke the next morning. We went downtown to check on repairs for the frame of one of her paintings. She was able to make the decisions on that.

At about 7:15 May 7th, with no suggestion from me, she said she needed to get up. I waited breakfast but decided to eat alone. When I was about done eating at 9:00 she came to the kitchen. We went to the hardware store after she ate and she stayed in the yard with me awhile as I did some work. She went to the computer with me in the afternoon and proof read some of the notes I had written. She made some suggestions for changes. I gladly made some of the changes and told her why I disagreed with one or two.

There was some talk when we woke May 8th, and she dressed with no help from me.

I asked May 9th if she wanted to do the walk out front. Ten or fifteen minutes later she asked if I was ready to go. She went to the computer about 8:30 PM and spent about an hour and a half proof reading a fifteen page brief of the notes I wrote about her illness. She thinks it makes her look bad. I tell her it shows how much she has improved.

I am not sure when I have felt worse than when I woke May 11th. She got to the kitchen soon after I finished breakfast. Both of us were better by lunch time. We did the walk out front in the afternoon. I called a friend whose husband has problems similar to Helen's. She told me he is not able to do many of the things Helen does.

When we woke May 12th I asked what time it was and she told me in a very clear voice. She started sobbing soon after that. She was awake when I went back at 8:30. I flashed the ceiling light on several times. She told me to stop it. We did the walk out front in the mid afternoon and I took her to the ladies' meeting which started at 7:00 PM.

I was awake May 13th when she turned on the light to see what time it was. There was some small talk. She was in good spirits. She dressed without my help and got to the kitchen at 9:25. She said I ate cereal. I asked how she knew and she said she did not see the frying pan out. Lunch and dinner at home went OK. We watched gospeel music on TV that night.

I worked in the yard some the morning of May 17th. When I went in to prepare lunch she was very low, but did the usual to help prepare lunch. When I quit the yard work about 5:00 she made two or three comments which told me she was better.

May 18th was the day of the ladies' luncheon. I told her one of us must prepare the dish for the church dinner before she leaves for the luncheon. She usually does most of that. After she ate I got out the things for the dinner dish and we prepared it together. Then we made the bed and I took her to the luncheon.

She woke me at 3:40 AM May 19th and said she heard a noise in the kitchen. I found I had not turned off the oven which we used to prepare dinner. It had been on more than twelve hours. I made the same mistake about a year ago and she heard it in the wee hours of the morning as she did just now. Her voice was so natural it sounded like it did years ago. I told her that and she said "I don't know about that". She went to sleep but I could not. I got up at 4:40 and read. I started reading Romans 8. I never got past verses I and 2. Then I went back to bed and to sleep. In the afternoon I suggested a walk out front or a drive up Scenic 7. She stood up in about five minutes and said " I guess we'd better take a drive". I asked where she wanted to go and she did not say, so I drove to Iron Mountain Park. We stopped there for awhile.

I tried to joke with her about 12:15 by asksing her if lunch was ready. I knew she could not prepard it alone. Then I told her what was available and asked what she wanted. After several minutes she said a turkey sandwich. She was oh so quiet. It was obvious she was hurting—not physical pain, but that sad feeling of not being able to do what she wanted to do. There have been so many days like that recently. I am concerned, but what can I do? We did the walk out front. I told her again it would be so wonderful if we could communicate.

She was ready for breakfast at 9:25 May 24th with no help from me. She asked what I ate and I told her. She chose the same. I needed to go downtown after lunch and I suggested going by the hospital to see a friend even though I had some reservations about that. The lady had both legs amputated recently, and she could not talk. I was pleased with how much Helen talked with the husband.

I did not help her May 26th but she was ready to eat at 9:00 and she fried her own bacon and egg. After she did the bike ride May 30th I said she dressed this morning with no help from me. She said "It took me long enough to do it". After dinner we had devotions together and I brought up some things that happened at the hospital which she did not remember. We had a lengthy talk about some things that happened at the hospital and about which I had a bad attitude. I believe I am now able to forgive these people. We played a game of UpWords after that. We had more serious two way conversation than we have had in a long time.

I asked June 1st if she was taking her Zoloft regularly. She said she had been out about a week. I should watch that closer. I wonder if that is why she has been so low the last few days. I spent a big part of the evening at the computer because she was so quiet.

When I woke about 6:30 June 2nd I could see she was awake, but she said nothing. I decided to see what she would do. She went to sleep again without saying one word, and I remained silent. She called me about 9:00. I handed her part of her underclothes, and I walked out. She came to the kitchen soon after that. She said good morning so low I could hardly hear it. I said nothing. My idea was to try to get her to see what she is doint to both of us. I just sat in the chair and watched her prepare her breakfast. When she started to sit down I said if she wanted anything to drink she could pour it.

She poured more orange juice. When she started toward the chair I motioned to the bike, and she did the back porch routine. Then I said "let's make the bed" and we did that together without either of us saying a word. When I mentioned salmon for dinner she said she did not know how to cook it. There was considerable talk after we went to bed. Some of that was serious and some was just small talk. She seemed surprised when I said her voice sounder more normal and like she sounded before she got sick.

We went to the grocery the next day and when we got back she said she was tired.

She talked a little when we woke June 6th. When she got up about 9:00 she commented that I did not take her orange juice to her. I had forgotten it. She started toward the bedroom about 10:00 and I aked what she was up to. She said she was going to make the bed, so I helped her.

There was considerable talk before we got up June 7th. I said I had not heard the school bus go by. She reminded me school was out.

She got to the bathroom about 8:20 June 8th, and got to the kitchen about 9:00 with no help from me. I tried to talk with her about lunch time, but she was silent. I broke down again. We did the walk out front in the afternoon.

I helped her start dressing June 12th and she said she did not have a dress. I disputed that. We had another quiet dinner out after church, and then went home. I did the laundry last night and put it in the dryer after we got home. We took it out about 2:00 and she carried some of it to the closet. When I went back there I saw she had fallen, and was on the floor. She said she fell when she started to pick up something. She did not appear to be hurt. She had some pain in the knee later, but nothing serious. At 10:45 she asked for ice cream. That was good to hear, as she so seldom asks for anything like that. When I bring out something to eat other than meal time she usually complains, but then eats it.

Before we got up June 15th she reminded me that was the day of the Christian women's luncheon.

She dressed June 16th and prepared her breakfast except I prepared her toast. She ate, put her dishes in the dishwasher, and did the back porch routine. This was finished about 10:00. Then we sat on the porch awhile before making the bed.

At about 4:00 PM June 18th I mention what we could have for dinner or we could go out. About ten or fifteen minutes later she said "I guess we'd better have the chicken".

When she got up June 20th she said she did not know what to put on, but she dressed with no help from me. She prepared her breakfast except I prepared her toast. Then at about 2:30 I asked if she wanted to do the walk out front.

She said nothing, but moved around in her chair. I helped her up and we did the walk.

The next day she asked what I ate for breakfast. I said saussage and egg. She said she wanted the same if I would prepare it for her. I did it.

She was awake at 6:00 June 28th and with no encouragement from me was up, dressed, and ready to eat at 7:45. She chose her breakfast quickly and it was great to eat breakfast with her. She has been very silent for several days, but shows signs of being better. While I was getting dinner she started crying that she did not know how to do something. I told her I was doing it and I did not like for her to imply I could not do it. I broke down. That was not nice of me.

She got to the kitchen at 9:55 July 1st. She noticed I had eaten a waffle and chose the same. We worked together to prepare it.

She was standing by her closet at 9:30 July 2nd, but not dressed. I went back at 10:20 and helped her start dressing. I did about two hours work in the yard after lunch. She told me that was too much. There was very limited talk as we ate dinner at home. If only we could have some communications. Years ago I never dreamed I could live in the same house with her and be so lonely. Well, really, she is not the same lady she was then.

When we woke July 5th she was better than I can remember in a long time.

She was like my wife of years ago. She was in the bathroom before 8:00 and ready to eat with me about 9:00. We went to the grocery after eating, and she was tired when we left the store.

When she woke the next day she was in fair shape, but nothing comparable to the day before. However, there was considerable two way conversation for the second consecutive day.

In the evening of July 8th we went to the computer to view a DVD of the Bible we got recently. She seemed interested, but had very little to say.

As of mid afternoon July 10th she had said practically nothing. I told her how it hurts me when we have no communication. After the evening church service I went to sleep in the chair about 9:15 and woke about 11:00. At that time she talked with me briefly in a very normal tone of voice.

We woke about 6:00 July 11th and she talked in a very normal tone of voice. We went back to sleep and when we woke about 7:00 she was in tears. I reminded her we were to have our pictures made and suggested she put on one of her nicer dresses. She said she did not know what it would be. I helped her start dressing.

She was ready to eat at 8:30 July 12th with no help from me.

I reminded her at 9:15 July 13th that Helen A. had requested she return her phone call. Helen A. had invited her to play scrabble with her at 4:00 this afternoon. Helen told me she did not see how she could do it. In my opinion there was no reason she could not. She was ready for breakfast about 10:00. After the usual routine we put together the dish for tonight's church dinner which we cooked later in the day.

After lunch July 16th I said something about going out and doing something different. She did not reply. I went to sleep in the chair and she woke me about 2:30. She got up and indicated, but did not say, she wanted to go. Then she said I needed to get gas, which I had forgotten. I mentioned three places we could go and she would not choose. We went to Petit Jean State Park for dinner. She seemed to enjoy the trip and there was a limited amount of two way conversation.

We had a pleasant breakfast together July 17th and it was not necessary for me to help her dress. I asked her to go to the porch and look at some work I had done getting ready to paint the railing. She was a painter, but I am not.

She made a few comments and seemed to agree with my ideas. There was more than the usual talk in the evening.

I suggested she look over some notes I had written for a counseling session by telephone with Focus on the Family. She was unhappy with some of the things I had written. I told her again both of us need help. I have tried to get her to go for counseling, but she is not willing.

I took her to the ladies' luncheon. She was extremely silent and told me nothing about the meeting.

It was late when I looked in July 23rd and saw her standing by her closet. I literally forced her to let me start dressing her, and then I walked out. She came out for breakfast about 10:30.

Dinner out after church July 24th continued the deadly silence. When we got to the car after eating I told her I did not know how much longer I can live under these circumstances. I told her not to be surprised any morning to find I have died in my sleep because I have nothing to live for. After we got home I asked if there was anything she was interested in the two of us doing in the future. She never said a word.

I had someone in the office at 10:00 July 27th and she went to the kitchen while he was here. In the evening we spent twenty or thirty minutes watching the DVD of the Bible.

I decided not to force her to get up July 31st and see what she would do. That was a mistake. We missed Sunday school.

As we were watching the 700 Club they mentioned a certain author who would be on later. We had seen him at conventions and sold his books when we were with Successful Living. I remembered him well, but she could not remember him.

I went in about 8:55 and helped her start dressing, and then walked out. She dressed with no further help from me, ate, and did the bike ride. We sat on the porch awhile and then made the bed. After dinner I mentioned going to the grocery. About 7:00 she asked if I was ready to go to the store. While on the way to the grocery we decided to go on a short trip to see the scenery and then we went to the grocery. It was a pleasant evening.

After the church service August 3rd I stopped the car at the foot of the drive and we did the walk out front without walking down or up the steep drive. She is so much better than she was a year ago.

It was almost noon when she finished breakfast August 12th. In the evening I brought up the subject of some of the racial things I saw when I was a child and as a young adult. She talked with me about that. We grew up in different parts of the country, and I think some of the things I said shocked her.

Getting her up in time for Sunday school August 7th was a major job. Breakfast was silent. There was a limited amount of conversation as we ate after church. There was more interesting two way conversation after we got home. That was great.

She dressed the next day with no help from me, and prepared her own breakfast except I buttered her toast.

The next day she came to the other room where I was and asked what time it was. Her watch showed the same time as mine. I think she was just bored sitting in the chair.

At about 12:00 noon the next day I sat down in the chair and asked what she wanted for lunch. She told me in about half an hour. In the evening I watered the lawn by moving the sprinkler to several places in the yard. Then she asked me if I had shut off the water. I had forgotten it.

Soon after breakfast we went to the grocery. I went to the computer after we put away the groceries. She called me and said she did not know what to do for lunch. I showed her the choices. As we were eating I suggested a certain trip and eating at a certain restaurant. About an hour later I asked what she wanted to do this afternoon. She said she thought we were going to Queen Willelmina State Park. I said I mentioned it but since she did not reply we had not talked about it. We left soon and had dinner at the park. We had a nice trip, but she was tired when we got back. I continue to believe a trip like that occasionally is good for both of us.

August 14th started off all too typical of Sunday mornings. In the afternoon she agreed to go for counseling.

When she got to the kitchen August 15th she saw the waffle iron out and rather quickly said she wanted a waffle. I prepared it for her. I was near the breaking point. About 1:00 she asked what we were doing for lunch, and I told her to go to the kitchen and see what was available. She chose something quicker than she usually does, and lunch went well. When I asked her to choose what she wanted for dinner she seemed to be choosing pink salmon and then she asked what we would have with it. I told her the vegetables were in the freezer and the closet. She made the choices. Dinner went very well. We made her impossible pie after dinner.

I forced her to get up at 8:00 August 16th. I told her I was going to the grocery and I expected her to be dressed when I got back. When I got back she had just finished eating. Then she made the bed and did the back porch routine. Dinner at home went quite well, but it was silent. After dinner we watched the DVD of the Bible.

When we woke about 7:00 August 17th she was more like she was years ago. While we were eating breakfast together she reminded me this was the day of the ladies' luncheon.

When she got to the kitchen August 18th she asked how long it would take to make a waffle. I prepared it for her. About 12:00 I told her I was about to call certain people and asked if she wanted to be in on the call. She did not answer my question, but asked if she had any breakfast. I told her she ate a waffle and we went out to lunch soon after that. After dinner we spent about forty-five minutes watchidng and listening to the Bible on DVD. Then I got out the church picture directory to find a man whose name I could not remember. It has been a better day.

She made some good choices when we went to the grocery August 19th even though she was very slow. I tried to get her on the phone when I was talking with my counselor, but her silence said no.

She dressed August 21st with no help from me. She was in the kitchen at 8:15, and we had a very pleasant breakfast together. It was a much better start for Sunday. After the evening service I encouraged her to do some things on the computer which would have been so simple to her before her illness. She was hesitant, but she did some things. This has been one of our best days recently and yesterday was so bad.

She seemed much better August 22nd and was ready to eat at 8:30. She was so sad again at lunch time. Dinner at home was another time of no communications. She had nothing to say. After dinner we spent considerable time watchindg the Bible on DVD and were both more relaxed adfter that.

When we woke about 7:00 August 23rd she said we could not lay there all day. I said she should get up and eat with me, but I did not force her to get up. She got up with no help from me and was in the kitchen at 8:05. She was silent, but we had a pleasant meal together. We had a pleasant lunch at home and then went to the grocery.

I went back at 9:05 August 29th and found her standing by the closet. I forced her to let me start dressing her, and then she finished and got to the kitchen at 9:50. She prepared her breakfast. Lunch and dinner at home were disasters and I was in bad shape. After dinner I told her I was going to the computer to work on something else, but if she wanted to watch the Bible on DVD to come in. Before I started the other she was at the computer with me. We watched the book of Psalms for about forty-five minutes and it was amazing how both of our attitudes changed.

We went to the Carven Gardens on the south side of Hot Springs September 1st. It was a wonderful tour, but she was so tired when we got home. We discussed this and decided it is probably better to do something like this occasionally even though she gets tired so easy.

I got back from the men's breakfast about 9:30 and she finished breakfast just before 12:00. Then I showed her how to prepare some pork ribs I planned to cook for dinner. She prepared them as I showed her every little detail. As

I have said before this just cannot be. Am I showing my wonderful wife who was such a great cook how to do anything in the kitchen? No, it just cannot be.

September 3rd I brought up some very serious things I believe may have contributed to her illness. She told me some things that happened before our marriage that she had not told me before. I told her she has grieved over that much too long, and she should forget about it. I believe she has, at times, remembered these things and then at other times burried them so deeply she believed it never happened.

She talked more than usual when we joined friends at a restaurant Sunday, September 4th. Then we went home and made a pie to take to the church picnic dinner before the evening servicee.

When we woke September 8th I asked her to get up and eat with me, but said I would not wait too long to eat with her. She was ready to eat at 8:30 and we had a pleasant breakfast together.

The next few days were not too different. I did some painting on the porch September 13thand after I worked about an hour and a quarter she came out and asked if I should not take a break. It has been a better day.

I got to bed before she did September 15th. I heard a noise in the bathroom and found she had fallen when she started to get off the stool. I helped her up and she did not appear to be injured. There were no injuries that showed up later.

September 16th we took a cruse on the lake with friends. There were 37 of us on the boat. When we walked back to the car from the boat she was very weak.

Through the years I have noticed many elderly people who are not able to leave their homes, or who spend so much time in hospitals. I have tried to see the two of us attend regular church services, and get out for a few other things. I believe this has been a big part of the reason Helen has improved so much. I am not saying this as an authority, but as an observation from our experience over the last three years plus.

Sunday morning I insisted she get up at 7:30. When she got up she fell and "landed" in a well padded chair sitting near her side of the bed. She was not hurt. It was scarey because this is the second time she has fallen in the last few days. When we got home after church I read some, and then showed her the book I was reading. There was a limited amount of two way conversation about this. Then we went out on the porch and looked at the painting I did yesterday. This led to more talk.

The next day she went for her first counseling session. The counselor, a PhD who has my greatest confidence, said she did not believe Helen had Altzheimer's because people who have that do not make the improvement Helen has made. That was good news for both of us. For dinner we tried the veggie burger recommended by her MD to help her cholesterol. We agreed that was not an ideal meal.

As we were sitting on the porch September 20th I mentioned some work I needed to do there in addition to the painting I recently finished. She looked over it very closely and I believe she was thinking clearly. She made a few comments. I believe such things are helpful to her because she loved such things before her illness. I said we need to buy a new table cloth for the umberlla table on the porch. She said we had two or three. She went to her studio room and found them quickly. I am sure she had not seen them since before her illness started more than three years ago. That is encouraging.

I helped her start dressing the next day and she finished . When I brought in some things from the yard I had moved to paint the porch she had some good ideas about how to rearrange things. I took her to the monthly ladies' luncheon. When I picked her up she had come out of the club to meet me because the meeting was over earlier than usual. As we were watching the 700 Club I received a very unusual, and undersireable, phone call. After we shut off the TV she asked what the call was about and I told her.

She called at 9:05 and said she did not know what to put on. I told her what to put on, but did not go back because I wanted to see what she would do. She called again in about fifteen minutes. I went back and helped her start dressing, and then I walked out. Then it was the old routine. She was so quiet. I broke again. I reminded her again how lonely I get when I am forced to live "alone" in the same house with her. That was not nice of me, but oh how it hurts.

We received a notice about a surprise 80th birthday party for an out of state friend. We will not be able to attend but I insisted she write something on a birthday card for him. She said "I can't" and I told her she could. She did. After that I could see signs she seemed to feel better.

After church Sunday she told me where she wanted to eat. She does not do that often. In the afternoon we listened to the second in a series of tapes we enjoy.

She had her second counseling appointment September 26th. The counselor said she is coming back. She made some choices about what we had for dinner at home.

She was not talking and was almost in tears when we woke September 28th. She was up in time to eat with me about 8:30.

She is not where I would like to see her, but she is so much better. What should I expect? We have both lived long lives, but who wants to get to the point they can do nothing? Or who wants to "check out"? We listened to another of the tapes on the book of Daniel.

She got up and dressed October 2nd with no help from me. That is great. The day went good except there was so little communicationn. If only we could discusss certain things and make plans.

We had a series of meetings at the church October 3rd through October 5th at 9:00 AM and 6:30 PM. She was up each morning in time to go to the 9:00 AM services. Both of us were helped by these meetings. It was three better days.

She said she had nothing to put on October 8th. I said her clothes were in the usual place and I made no effort to help her. She came out ready to eat about 9:30. When she started to eat cereal I asked why she bought the special diet for cholsterol. Then she got out the eggbeater and I prepared it for her.

She was up and ready to eat October 9th earlier than usual, even for Sunday, with no help from me.

She had her third counseling session October 3rd. She was alone with the lady counselor, and she told me nothing about it. She did seem better after the session.

She was ready to eat earlier than usual October 16th even though I did not insist on her getting up. The day went very good compared to most days recently.

I took her orange juice in about 8:00 October 20th. Other than turning on the overhead light I did nothing to insist on her getting up. She went to the bathroon at 8:50, and I insisted that she start dressing. I did very little to help her dress. She finished eating and washing the dishes about 11:30. Then at my suggestion she did the bike ride. We sat on the porch awhile and then made the bed. We attended a meeting in the afternoon where the medicare program was explained.

The next day I told her I had to take some things to the dump. I insisted she get up earlier than usual. We ate together at 8:30. The trip downtown went OK, but she could not talk with me about anything. I broke down again.

She was whimpering about the time she woke October 23rd. I insisted she get up and then I walked out. I forced her to start dressing and then I walked out again. She used the old story about not knowing what to put on. I asked what she wanted to eat and she would not (or could not?) tell me. I fianally told her I would prepare my breakfast, and she could prepare hers if she would not tell me what she wanted. Then she prepared her cereal.

We saw her counselor October 24th. Did I say her counselor? The counselor spent more time with me than with Helen. She gave us a good report about Helen.

After she ate breakfast I made a call to her doctor's office to talk about the diet she is on for cholesterol. She was on the phone, but said practically nothing. Her counselor had suggested a change in her medication. When I mentioned that I was told the doctor should see her before he would change it. She cried as she agreed to make the appointment. What would it be like to have pleasant communication and lengthy conversations with her again?

We attended the Couples Club dinner October 29th.

We were awake at 5:30 October 31st. I went back to sleep, but she said she did not. We ate together about 9:00 and she did the back porch routine.

The next day I had a client in the office so I did not try to get her up early. She finished breakfast about 11:30. We went to the grocery in the afternoon and she seemed considerably better.

She dressed without my help November 3rd and ate about 10:00. We went downtown for a bonescan prescribed by her doctor. We watched the Bible on DVD after dinner. Then I suggested watching a DVD by Dr James Dobson. Then I said since we just watched the DVD it might be better to see Dr Dobson's later. After considerable hesitation she decided to watch it then. It has been a better day. AND three years ago today one doctor told me he would give her four to six weeks and then "let her go".

We got flue shots November 10th. We went to the grocery together and I took her to the monthly ladies' meeting at church in the evening.

Thursday night the electronic door opener on our garage door went out. We have an appointment to have it repaired Monday. It was raining as we walked out to the car to go to church. I was holding her arm with one hand and the umberlla in the other hand. She fell as we were walking down the steps. She was not injured.

I made a waffle yesterday using the low cholosterol recipe. She ate one yesterday and chose another one today. I prepared her dinner a little early and I went to a men's dinner at out church. She was eating when I left and I was gone a little over two hours. When I returned she had put her dishes in the dishwasher and was sitting in her usual chair. I hate to leave her alone and do not do it often. She seemed to be OK, and I certainly enjoyed the men's meeting.

This is missionary weekend at out church. Saturday night we visited at the home of friends who had missionaries who serve with Wycliffe Bible Translators. When I insisted she get up November 22nd she said she did not know what to put on. As I walked out I said "so what's new"? I went back and helped her start dressing.

Alzheimer's, Depression and Dementia

When she said she did not know what to put on Thanksgiving day I told her saying that or saying "I can't" was vulgar and she should watch her language. When she came out about 9:15 she was wearing what I suggested. We had Thanksgiving dinner at the home of friends.

There was nothing too different about most of the next day. When the 700 Club was over at 11:00 PM I shut off the TV and leaned back in the chair and said nothing. After a long time she called my name and I said nothing. Then at 11:30 she asked if I wanted to go to bed. I said I was waiting to see if she would speak to me. Her voice was loud and clear—very normal. She said nothing after that. This is so discouraging.

There was more than the usual two way conversation November 30th. It was a much better day. It is amazing, but should be no surprise, how much her condition changes my feelings. When she is better I feel so much better.

The next day we had an appointment with a new MD recommended by her counselor. She started the old "I can't" and I told her she would. I got the Zoloft bottle to show the new doctor and found it was empty. She said she had been out several days. I should have watched that closer. I called the pharmacy for a refill. It appears she has been out a little less than a week and she has been so low the last few days.

December 4th started off bad. She finally put on a nice two piece outfit after I insisted she not wear either of two dresses she had worn so often lately. Breakfast was in near silence. When we got to the resturant after church it was hard for me to hold back the tears. We had such a wonderful marriage prior to her illness.

We attended the annual Christmas dinner for our Sunday school class December 9th. There were about forty-five people present. She seemed to enjoy it, and was better when we got home. It has been a better day.

We had an appointment with her counselor December 12th. I am not sure whether the person being counseled is Helen or me.

She dressed December 13th with almost no help from me. Lunch and dinner at home went OK, and we went to the grocery in the afternoon.

She seemed to be in good shape when she woke December 18th, but when she got up she started the old "I can't". There was considerable talk before she got up, but after she got up she was so silent. The silence continued through breakfast, church, and lunch. There was more communication after we got home.

Since this is the day of the ladies' luncheon I insisted she eat breakfast earlier. She finished breakfast about 9:45, and then we made the bed. I took her to the luncheon. After we went to bed her voice was very clear.

I woke about 4:45 AM December 22nd and went to the bath room. When I went back to bed she was awake and we talked about the pleasant conversation we had last night. I think she slept some after that. I was so keyed up about last night I slept very little more, if any. We ate breakfast together and finished about 9:45. I did not suggest it, but she rinsed the dishes and put them in the dishwasher. Then we made the bed. She did not talk much at the table, but she smiled a lot. Things do look better. I believe our Lord is working. Yesterday I showed her a Christmas letter I had written and asked her opinion. It is late. She suggested a change or two. Today I thought of a change I wanted to make. After I made the changes I printed one copy and showed it to her. She said "I think it's all right". There was considerable two way conversation in the late evening.

December 24th started off with me in worse shape than her. I did very little to help her dress. We attended the Christmas Eve service at our church which started at 6:00 PM. It was a wonderful service, as it always is.

Can this really be Christmmas? This is the fourth Christmas since Helen got sick. I have become all too familiar with what I have heard about Thanksgiving and Christmas being so lonely for certain people. Now I know from personal experience. We had only one service at the church today. That was at 10:30 with no Sunday school or evening service. We ate the noon meal at a nice resturant downtown where the food was great. But we were alone and there was practically no communication between us. And this was Christmas? I came to the computer about 9:30 PM to write this. I had just finished reading some pretty heavy stuff friends sent with their Christmas card. Helen was reading that when I went to the computer. That resulted in some communication for which I am thankful.

She dressed with very little help from me December 26th, but she was so silent. Lunch was almost as silent as breakfast. I worked in the yard an hour or so in the late afternoon. I went in the house to put water on something I was cooking and found she had already done it. I told her that was good.

Before she got up December 29th I received a call from a friend inviting us to have dinner at her home at 5:30 today. I said nothing to Helen about this call till we were eating lunch. I did this to see if she heard the call, or if she would say anything to me about it. When I mentioned it she said it was something about 5:30. I told her we were invited to have dinner at Joyce's home. When we got there we were pleasantly surprised to find two other couples we knew were there. Joyce had invited us because she knew yesterday was our wedding anniversary. While we were there several people told some interesting stories, and Helen laughed more than I had heard her laugh in a long time. I reminded her of this on the way home, and she did not say a word. I never heard her laugh again.

She had an appointment with her hair dresser at 10:30 December 30th, so she got up earlier than usual. She did her bike ride after lunch. She seems to feel better, but is so quiet. As mentioned above we were invited to eat with friends last night. After a delicious meal the hostess insisted we fill plates to take home for another meal. When we ate dinner the following day Helen said she was just not able to eat that much. I am really concerned because I wonder if the end is near. I have wondered about this before, but our Lord has left her here so far. Maybe He will continue to do so for some more time. As I remember she weighed about 154 pounds before she got sick. When she came home from the nursing home she weighed about 135 pounds. I insisted she get on the bathroom scales a couple of days ago and she weighed less than 120 pounds.

She was in no hurry to get up Dec 31st and did not seem to know what to put on. She said she had a pain in her stomach. I said she ate so little last night she was probably hungry. She got to the kitchen about 10:00 and ate a little more than usual. We usually eat a sandwich and fruit or pie at lunch. She chose a chicken sandwich for lunch and I brought out peach pie. She ate no more than a third of the sandwich and said she could eat no more. She ate the pie, but did not eat any of the crust. I brought out the remainder of the sandwich about 3:30. She began to cry and did not eat a bite of it. I asked her to help me make her imposible pie for the church dinner tonight. She did not really want to, but she went to the kitchen. She was so low all day. We had a pot luck dinner at the church, and saw the first half of the Ben Hur movie. The remainder of the movie will be shown later. She ate very little and was very quiet. She did talk with me a little after the movie.

January 1st, 2006 did not start off too different from the typical Sunday. I had to force her to start dressisng. I suggested she wear a certain outfit because she had worn the same two dresses so much recently. She finally came out wearing the outfit I suggested. We got to Sunday school a few minutes late.

I have seen cases where one is sick and they are confined to the house so long. This is probably unpreventable in some cases, and I certainly do not condem them for that. Even before Helen came home from the nursing home I tried to get her out as much as possible. A big part of what we did was attend our church as much as possible. We did various other things to try to make life as near normal as possible. There were many times when I felt the total responsibility was on me, and that added to the load. I believe this has been a wise decision. After church today we went out to eat and there was no big difference in the remainder of the day except there was no evening service at the church, due to the holidays.

After I wrote the above I asked her to read it and tell me what she thought about it. She spent ten or fifteen minutes studying it, and said she was in agreement. I mentioned a certain book of the Bible I wanted to listen to on DVD. She said "I feel awful" and went to the living room.

When she woke January 2nd she said her stomach hurt. I said she was probably hungry because she ate so little last night. We went through this same deal a few days ago. She was ready to eat about 9:00. She ate more cereal than she usually eats, but refused to eat toast. About 10:00 I asked if she wanted to help me make the bed or if she wanted me to make it. She helped me. I could have done it, but I thought it would be good for her to be out of the chair more. I received a call from a client who suggested we meet for lunch and discuss her taxes. Helen went with me and we had a nice meeting except she ate only about a third of a chicken sandwich. I took the remainder home and about 4:30 she ate about half of what was left. Dinner was at home, and she ate a fairly good meal. She said something just before I got dinner ready that caused me to think she was hungry.

After dinner I noticed her stomach was swollen. I asked if she wanted to go to the emergency room and she said no. I helped her walk to the bedroom at bedtime because I thought it might not be safe for her to try to walk alone. She has an appointment with an MD at 1:15 tomorrow. She said she had not had a bowel movement in two days, and indicated it may have been longer than that. I suggested she drink some prune juice and she did that.

We were awake at 4:00 AM January 3rd and again at 5:00. Her stomach was swolen and she had not had a bowell movement. I suggested she drink more prune juice, and she said not to give her as much as I gave her last night. She was not able to swallow all of it, and some of it came out of her mouth.

I cleaned her chin with a Kleenex. It was necessary for me to help her out of bed and to the bathroom. That was unusual. While setting on the stool she said she needed a shower. I helped her up, and it was very difficult to lift her. She did not seem to be able to do anything to get up by herself. She never got her shower cap on. She gripped the rod of the towel rack with both hands and held it very firmly. I grabbed her and tried to get her to the bed, but was unable to do so. She could not move by herself, and I was not able to get her back to the bed. I let her go gently to the floor. She did not fall. I called 911 and then massaged her heart. The para medics arrived soon.

I was told she was not able to breathe on her own. I knew she was gone, but was not willing to admit it. Shortly after we got to the hospital I was told Helen was dead.

So many people at the church, and others, have been so helpful during and after her long illness. I do not dare try to name them because I would not be able to name all of them.

This last paragraph is being written May 31st, 2006—hardly five months after her death. I am determined to make life as near normal as possible, but I know that without Helen life will never be normal again. Through the years I have heard many strange stories about things that happened to the survivor after the death of a spouse. It has come to the point I usually get a good night's sleep. Normally I wake about 6:30 in the morning. The night of May 23rd-24th I slept good till 5:30 AM when I woke as I heard Helen call my name. I did not see her clearly, but I heard her call my name very clearly and the tone of her voice was pleasant. That was all I heard.

Printed in the United States
128195LV00002BA/13-36/P